# ACTIVATING THE POWER OF THE BRAIN

# This is your brain on food

## DEPRESSION,ANXIETY,PTSD,ADHD, OCD AND MORE

## BY

# DR BEN JAPHETH

# TABLE OF CONTENT

# Chapter 2

# The Science of Nutritional Psychiatry

How food affects mood and mental health

Key nutrients for brain health

# Chapter 3

# Depression-Busting Foods

Foods that can palliate symptoms of depression

Recipes and meal plans

# Chapter 4

# Anxiety-Reducing Diet

Foods to help manage anxiety

Meal plans for anxiety

# Conclusion

The role of food in mental health

Encouragement for readers to take charge of
their diet and mental wellness

# INTR0DUCTION

# Why food matter for mental health

The Vital Connection: How Food Matters for Mental Health

Chronic inflammation has emerged as a common factor in various mental health disorders, including depression and schizophrenia. Diet is very important in modulating inflammation levels in the body. A diet high in processed foods, refined sugars, and unhealthy fats can promote inflammation, which could potentially play a role in the onset or worsening of mental health issues. On the other hand, a diet rich in fruits, vegetables, whole grains, and lean proteins provides antioxidants and anti-inflammatory compounds that can help mitigate the inflammatory response.

# Blood Sugar Regulation and Mood Stability

The impact of diet on blood sugar levels extends beyond physical health. Consuming foods with a high glycemic index—those that cause rapid spikes and fluctuation in blood sugar levels may result in mood swings, irritability and fatigue. These fluctuations are particularly problematic for individuals with conditions like bipolar disorder. Choosing complex carbohydrates, which release energy more steadily, helps maintain stable blood sugar levels and supports emotional equilibrium.

## The Social and Psychological Aspects of Eating

Food isn't just nourishment for the body; it's also a significant part of our social and cultural lives. Eating together with family and friends nurtures a feeling of connection and belonging, which are crucial for mental well-being. Additionally, the act of eating itself can be a pleasurable experience that contributes to the release of dopamine, a neurotransmitter associated with reward and pleasure.

However, it's important to note that the relationship between food and mental health is complex and multifaceted. While diet can play a pivotal role, it's not a singular solution for managing mental health conditions. Mental health is controlled by diverse elements, such as genetics, surroundings, and one's way of life, collectively shaping and impacting this outcome and access to proper care.

In the pursuit of holistic well-being, the significance of food for mental health cannot be overstated. The evidence pointing to the intricate links between diet and psychological well-being highlights the importance of making informed dietary choices. While further research is needed to fully comprehend the mechanisms underlying this relationship, there is little doubt that nurturing our bodies with a balanced and nutrient-rich diet can contribute positively to our mental health. Integrating nutritional considerations into mental health care could pave the way for more comprehensive approaches to managing and preventing mental health disorders.

## The Gut-Brain Connection

The Gut-Brain Connection: Unveiling the Intricate Link Between Your Gut and Mind

In the realm of human health, the interplay between various bodily systems has always intrigued researchers and medical professionals. One of the most remarkable and intricate connections to emerge in recent years is the gut-brain connection, a fascinating network that showcases the profound relationship between the gut and the brain. This connection has far-reaching implications for both physical and mental well-being, shedding light on how our digestive system communicates with and influences our cognitive and emotional states.

## A Bi-Directional Communication Superhighway

The gut-brain connection, often referred to as the gut-brain axis, is a complex and bi-directional communication pathway between the gastrointestinal tract and the central nervous system. This communication takes place through a combination of neural, hormonal, and immune mechanisms. The vagus nerve, a major nerve connecting the gut to the brain, serves as a crucial conduit for this exchange of information. Signals travel both from the gut to the brain and vice versa, influencing various aspects of our physiological and mental functioning.

## The Role of Gut Microbiota

At the heart of the gut-brain connection lies the gut microbiota, an intricate ecosystem of trillions of microorganisms inhabiting our digestive tract. These microorganisms, including bacteria, viruses, and fungi, collectively form a diverse and dynamic community that plays a pivotal role in our health. Recent research has revealed that the gut microbiota not only impacts digestion and nutrient absorption but also has a profound influence on our mood, behavior, and cognitive function.

The gut microbiota engages in a symbiotic relationship with the body, aiding in the breakdown of complex carbohydrates, producing certain vitamins, and supporting the immune system. Moreover, these microorganisms produce a wide array of metabolites and signaling molecules that can affect brain function. For instance, the gut microbiota produces neurotransmitters such as Serotonin and dopamine play crucial roles in the regulation of mood and emotions.

## Influence on Mental Health

The gut-brain connection has garnered considerable attention for its role in mental health.

A growing body of evidence indicates that disturbances in the gastrointestinal system microbiota, a condition known as dysbiosis, are associated with an increased risk of mental health disorders, including anxiety, depression, and even conditions like autism and schizophrenia. Researchers have observed altered patterns of gut microbiota composition in individuals with these conditions, highlighting the potential influence of gut health on brain function.

The production of neurotransmitters by gut bacteria, coupled with the impact of the gut microbiota on inflammation and immune response, further solidifies the link between gut health and mental health. Moreover, the gut-brain connection may explain why gastrointestinal symptoms often accompany mental health disorders, a phenomenon known as the "gut-brain axis dysfunction."

## Diet and the Gut-Brain Connection

One's diet significantly influences the makeup and variety of microorganisms in the gut microbiota. The foods we consume serve as fuel for these microorganisms, influencing their growth and activity. A diet rich in fiber, fruits, vegetables, and fermented foods can promote the growth of beneficial bacteria, supporting a healthy gut microbiota and potentially positively impacting mental health. On the other hand, a diet high in processed foods, added sugars, and unhealthy fats can lead to an imbalanced microbiota and potential negative effects on mood and cognition.

## Holistic Implications and Future Directions

The gut-brain connection has immense implications for both medical and holistic approaches to health care. Integrative strategies that consider the interplay between gut health, mental health, and overall well-being are gaining momentum. Medical professionals are increasingly exploring interventions such as probiotics and prebiotics, dietary changes, and even fecal microbiota transplantation to address mental health issues.

As research continues to unravel the complexities of the gut-brain connection, it opens doors to novel therapeutic avenues and preventive strategies. However, while the link is clear, it's essential to recognize that mental health is influenced by a multitude of factors, and the gut-brain connection is just one piece of the puzzle. Nonetheless, the emerging insights into this connection mark a promising step towards a more comprehensive understanding of human health and the potential for more holistic approaches to well-being.

# Chapter 1

# Understanding

# Mental Health Disorders

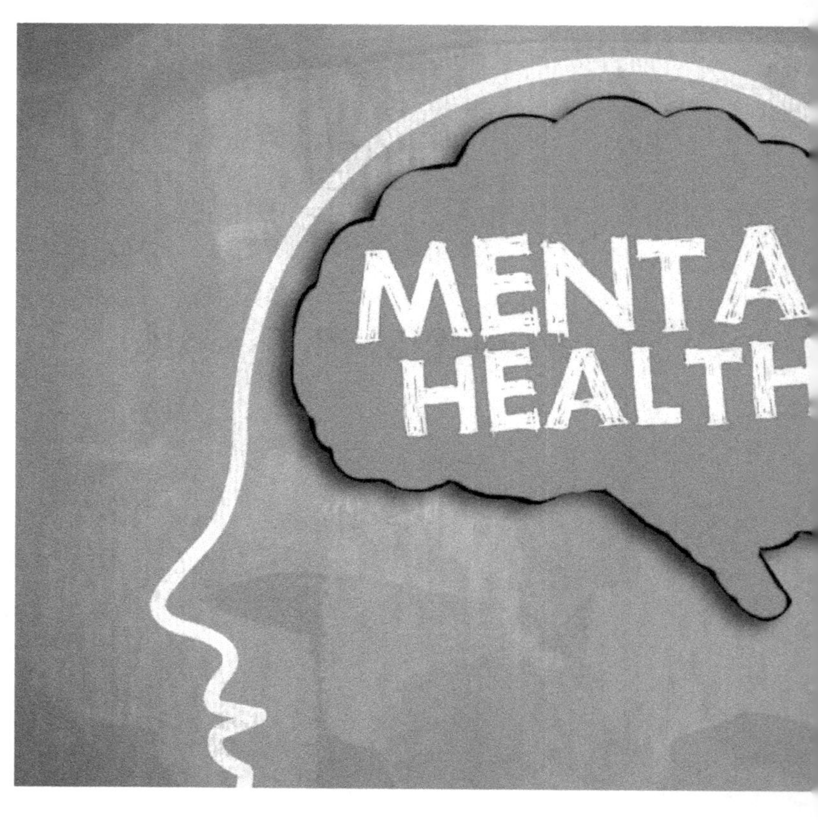
MENTA
HEALTH

# Navigating the Landscape of Mental Health: Understanding Depression, Anxiety, PTSD, ADHD, OCD, and More

In the realm of mental health, a diverse spectrum of conditions exists, each with its unique challenges and manifestations. From the depths of depression to the relentless grip of anxiety, and the complexities of conditions like PTSD, ADHD, and OCD, the human mind's intricacies are a landscape worth exploring. In this article, we'll provide a brief explanation of these conditions, shedding light on their core features and offering a glimpse into the lives of those affected.

## Depression: Unraveling the Weight of Emotional Darkness

In the vast landscape of human emotions, there exists a profound and complex territory known as depression. This mental health condition reaches far beyond mere sadness, casting a heavy shadow on the lives of those it touches. Often described as a relentless weight of emotional darkness, depression is a journey that warrants understanding, empathy, and a compassionate approach.

### The Depths of Despair

Depression is more than a passing mood or a temporary case of the blues.

It's characterized by persistent feelings of sadness, hopelessness, and a profound loss of interest or pleasure in activities that once sparked joy. While sadness is a natural emotion experienced by all, depression lingers like a fog, obscuring one's ability to see beyond it.

The experience of depression goes beyond mere emotions—it permeates physical sensations, thoughts, and behaviors. Fatigue, changes in sleep and appetite, difficulty concentrating, and even physical aches become unwelcome companions. A sense of isolation often accompanies depression, as individuals find it challenging to connect with others or explain the depth of their struggles.

## A Complex Tapestry of Causes

Depression should not be viewed as a manifestation of weakness, nor is it a matter of choice. It's a complex interplay of factors that include genetics, brain chemistry, hormonal imbalances, life experiences, and environmental influences. Traumatic events, loss, chronic stress, and major life changes can trigger or exacerbate depressive episodes.

The brain's intricate network of neurotransmitters, which regulate mood and emotion, plays a significant role in depression.

Imbalances in these chemical messengers can disrupt communication pathways, leading to the emotional turmoil that characterizes the condition.

### The Stigma Surrounding Depression

Despite the prevalence of depression—more than 264 million people worldwide experience it—stigma still surrounds the condition. Misconceptions that depression is a sign of weakness or can be "snapped out of" perpetuate misunderstandings. Such beliefs can hinder individuals from seeking help and contribute to their feelings of isolation.

### Seeking Light in the Darkness

Recovery from depression is possible, but it's not a linear path. Treatment often involves a combination of approaches tailored to the individual's needs. Psychotherapy, such as cognitive-behavioral therapy (CBT), can provide tools to challenge negative thought patterns and develop coping strategies. Medication, such as antidepressants, can help restore neurotransmitter balance.

Support from loved ones is essential in the journey toward recovery. A listening ear, empathy, and nonjudgmental presence can provide solace to those grappling with depression. Encouraging professional help and offering companionship during treatment can make a significant difference.

**Breaking the Silence**

Increasing awareness and open dialogue about depression are crucial steps toward stigmatization. It's vital to recognize that depression doesn't discriminate; it can impact individuals of any age, gender, or background.

By fostering an environment of understanding, we can create spaces for

encouraging people to openly discuss their experiences without the fear of being judged is important.

If you or someone you know is struggling with depression, remember that reaching out for assistance is a display of strength, not a display of weakness.

Professional support can provide guidance, tools, and a sense of hope on the journey toward healing. Together, through compassion and knowledge, we can lighten the weight of emotional darkness and pave the way for brighter days ahead.

<u>**Anxiety: The Unrelenting Worry that Clouds the Mind**</u>

In the intricate tapestry of human emotions, anxiety stands as a formidable thread, weaving its way into the lives of millions worldwide. Far more than the occasional nervousness that everyone experiences, anxiety is an unrelenting and often overwhelming state of worry that can grip the mind and body. Understanding this complex mental health condition is essential for fostering empathy, providing support, and promoting a brighter path for those caught in its grip.

<u>**The Anatomy of Anxiety**</u>

Anxiety is a multifaceted emotional state characterized by excessive worry, apprehension, and a sense of unease. It goes beyond the usual pre-event jitters or concerns about the future, often presenting itself without an apparent trigger. Anxiety can manifest as physical symptoms, such as racing heart, trembling, sweating, and gastrointestinal distress, further adding to the distress of those who experience it.

While anxiety can serve as a protective mechanism in certain situations, such as alerting us to potential dangers, its intensification can become problematic. Anxiety disorders involve a chronic pattern of excessive worry and fear that it disrupts everyday life, relationships, and overall well-being.

**The Spectrum of Anxiety Disorders**

Anxiety disorders manifest in different forms, each with its distinct features:

Generalized Anxiety Disorder (GAD): This involves pervasive and excessive GAD may feel restless, on edge, and find it challenging to control their worries.

Social Anxiety Disorder: Individuals with social anxiety encounter profound apprehension and discomfort in social situations. They often fear being judged or embarrassed, leading to avoidance of gatherings or interactions.

Panic Disorder: Characterized by sudden and intense episodes of fear known as panic attacks, panic disorder can lead to physical symptoms like chest pain, shortness of breath, and a feeling of impending doom.

Specific Phobias: These involve an intense and irrational fear of specific Objects, situations, or activities like heights, flying, or spiders can trigger specific phobias.

Obsessive-Compulsive Disorder (OCD): OCD combines intrusive thoughts (obsessions) with repetitive behaviors or mental rituals (compulsions) aimed at alleviating anxiety. It often leads to a cycle of distress and compulsive actions.

Post-Traumatic Stress Disorder (PTSD): Following a traumatic event, PTSD can cause intrusive memories, nightmares, flashbacks, and emotional numbness.

## The Weight of Unrelenting Worry

Living with anxiety is akin to carrying an invisible weight, with worries cascading through the mind like a torrential rain. Simple tasks can become monumental challenges as the mind becomes consumed by apprehension and fear. Anxiety has a way of distorting reality, magnifying potential threats and eroding the ability to find calmness or peace.

The persistent nature of anxiety can be exhausting, leading to physical and emotional fatigue.

Sleep disturbances, irritability, and difficulties in concentration are common companions to those grappling with anxiety. Relationships may strain as communication becomes hindered by the unending cycle of worry.

## Support and Healing

Acknowledging anxiety's impact is the first step toward finding relief and healing. Seeking support from mental health professionals, such as therapists or counselors, can provide tools to manage anxiety. Cognitive-behavioral therapy (CBT) is particularly effective in addressing anxious thought patterns and replacing them with healthier ones.

Engaging in relaxation techniques, mindfulness practices, regular exercise, and a balanced diet can also contribute to managing anxiety. Building a strong supportive network of friends, family, and peers who comprehend and share empathy.

with the challenges of anxiety can be immensely helpful.

**Breaking the Silence**

Raising awareness and promoting open conversations about anxiety are essential for stigmatization.

Recognizing that anxiety is a prevalent and legitimate struggle helps create an environment where those affected feel safe seeking help and sharing their experiences.

If you or someone you know is wrestling with anxiety, remember that you're not alone, and help is available.

By extending a hand of empathy, patience, and understanding, we can offer a beacon of light to guide individuals through the unrelenting worry and toward a path of healing and hope.

**PTSD: Reliving Trauma's Echoes and the Journey to Healing**

In the intricate landscape of human emotions, the echoes of trauma can reverberate long after the events have passed.

Post-Traumatic Stress Disorder (PTSD) is a complex and deeply impactful mental health condition that arises from experiencing or witnessing traumatic events. It casts a long shadow over the lives of those affected, but with understanding, support, and the right resources, a path to healing can be forged.

## Unraveling the Trauma

PTSD emerges in the aftermath of a traumatic event that threatens an individual's physical or emotional well-being. This can include experiences like combat, accidents, natural disasters, sexual assault, abuse, or even life-threatening medical procedures. Instead of fading into the past, the memories of such events become trapped in the mind, persistently intruding on daily life.

## The Hallmarks of PTSD

At the heart of PTSD are symptoms that encompass a wide range of emotional, cognitive, and physiological responses.

Intrusive memories, flashbacks, nightmares, and distressing thoughts are common, often making the individual feel as if they are reliving the traumatic event.

Avoidance behaviors, such as avoiding reminders of the trauma or numbing emotions, are used as coping mechanisms to shield against the overwhelming distress.

Hyperarousal symptoms from another facet of PTSD, characterized by heightened startle responses, irritability, difficulty concentrating, and a constant sense of being on edge. These symptoms create a state of perpetual alertness, as if the individual is bracing for another traumatic event.

## The Isolation of Trauma

The impact of PTSD extends beyond its symptoms, often causing a profound sense of isolation. People with PTSD may find it challenging to explain their experiences or may feel that others cannot understand the depth of their emotional turmoil. This isolation can strain relationships and contribute to feelings of loneliness and alienation.

# The Path to Healing

While the echoes of trauma may seem insurmountable, there is hope in the journey to healing. Seeking professional help is a crucial step, as therapists experienced in trauma-focused therapies can provide tools to manage symptoms and address the underlying emotional wounds. Cognitive-behavioral therapies (CBT) and eye movement desensitization and reprocessing (EMDR) are among the effective therapeutic approaches used to assisting individuals in processing and managing traumatic memories. Support from loved ones is vital, offering a safe space for individuals to share their experiences and emotions. Encouraging professional help and offering understanding can help create an environment conducive to healing.

## The Power of Resilience

Resilience is an integral part of the journey to recovery from PTSD. While the echoes of trauma may never fully dissipate, with time and appropriate treatment, their impact can be diminished. The path to healing is not linear—there will be ups and downs, but progress is possible.

It's important to acknowledge that each person's healing journey from trauma is unique, and there is no universally "correct" path to recovery. Patience, self-compassion, and a supportive network are essential companions on this journey.

## Fostering Understanding and Compassion

Raising awareness about PTSD is vital for breaking down the stigma that can surround this condition. It's crucial to recognize that trauma's echoes are not a sign of weakness but a reflection of the human mind's attempt to process and heal from deeply distressing events.

By fostering understanding, empathy, and open conversations about PTSD, we create a space where those affected feel seen and heard. With the right resources and a community of support, individuals can navigate the path to healing and reclaim their lives from the grasp of trauma's echoes.

## ADHD: Navigating the Challenge of Focus and Impulsivity

In a world bustling with stimuli and demands, the ability to maintain focus and control impulses is a valuable skill. For individuals with Attention-Deficit/Hyperactivity Disorder (ADHD), this task is often akin to navigating a complex labyrinth. ADHD is a disease that affects attention, impulse control, and executive functioning. Understanding the intricacies of ADHD is essential for fostering empathy and providing appropriate support to those facing its challenges.

The ADHD Spectrum

ADHD exists along a spectrum, with its symptoms manifesting differently in various individuals. The two primary subtypes are:

Predominantly Inattentive Presentation: Characterized by difficulties in sustaining attention, organization, and completing tasks. Individuals with this subtype may appear dreamy or forgetful, often losing track of details.

Predominantly Hyperactive-Impulsive Presentation: This subtype involves restlessness, impulsivity, and difficulty regulating impulses. People with this presentation may interrupt conversations, struggle with patience, and find it hard to sit still.

Combined Presentation: Some individuals exhibit a combination of inattentive and hyperactive-impulsive symptoms.

## The Impact on Daily Life

ADHD's effects extend beyond occasional lapses in attention. It can impact academic performance, work productivity, personal relationships, and self-esteem. Simple tasks can become monumental challenges as individuals struggle with organizing thoughts, managing time, and completing assignments.

Impulsivity, a hallmark of ADHD, can lead to decision-making without considering consequences. This can manifest as blurting out thoughts, acting without thinking, or engaging in risky behaviors. While impulsivity can have positive attributes, such as spontaneity, it can also cause difficulties in managing daily responsibilities.

### Neurobiological Underpinnings

ADHD's roots lie in neurobiological factors. Neurotransmitters like dopamine play a significant role in regulating attention and impulse control. In individuals with ADHD, there may be imbalances in these neurotransmitter systems, affecting the brain's ability to maintain attention and regulate impulses.

Genetics also contribute to ADHD risk. Family history of the disorder can increase the likelihood of its occurrence. Environmental factors, such as exposure to toxins during pregnancy, low birth weight, or premature birth, can also play a role.

## Navigating the Challenges

While ADHD presents challenges, it's important to remember that it also brings strengths. People with ADHD often possess creativity, energy, and the ability to think outside the box. Recognizing these qualities can help build self-esteem and resilience.

Managing ADHD involves a multimodal approach. Behavioral interventions, psychoeducation, and executive functioning skills training are integral components. Medication, such as stimulants or non-stimulants, can help regulate neurotransmitter levels and improve attention and impulse control.

## Support and Understanding

Support from family, friends, and educators is crucial for individuals with ADHD.

A structured environment, clear expectations, and positive reinforcement can help create a supportive framework. Flexibility, patience, and open communication are key to helping those with ADHD navigate challenges.

## Shattering Stigma

Raising awareness and dispelling misconceptions about ADHD is essential for shattering stigma. ADHD is not a result of laziness, lack of discipline, or poor parenting. All neurological conditions require understanding and support.

By fostering empathy, providing resources, and creating an inclusive environment, we can empower individuals with ADHD to navigate the challenge of focus and impulsivity, harness their unique strengths, and thrive in a world that celebrates diversity of thought and experience.

# OCD: The Unending Loop of Intrusive Thoughts and the Quest for Control

Within the intricate realm of the human mind, there lies a condition that casts individuals into an unending loop of intrusive thoughts, obsessions, and compulsions. Obsessive-Compulsive Disorder (OCD) is a complex mental health condition that can profoundly impact daily life. Understanding the nuances of OCD is crucial for fostering empathy, eradicating misconceptions, and supporting those who navigate its challenges.

## Understanding Obsessive-Compulsive Disorder

OCD is characterized by two intertwined components: obsessions and compulsions. Obsessions are intrusive and distressing thoughts, images, or urges that repeatedly infiltrate the mind. Compulsions are regular behaviors or mentally leads to alleviate anxiety which is caused by obsessions. Despite offering temporary relief, compulsions often fuel the cycle, leading to more intrusive thoughts and a heightened sense of distress.

# The Unrelenting Loop

Imagine being trapped in a cycle where unwanted thoughts are akin to unwelcome guests who refuse to leave. People with OCD grapple with a relentless cycle of intrusive thoughts that trigger intense anxiety. These thoughts can range from fears of contamination, harm to oneself or others, or disturbing religious or sexual imagery.

In an attempt to quell the anxiety caused by obsessions, individuals engage in compulsive behaviors. These rituals might involve washing hands excessively, checking locks multiple times, or mentally repeating certain phrases. However, these behaviors only offer fleeting relief, as the anxiety inevitably returns, perpetuating the cycle of obsession and compulsion.

## The Struggle for Control

At the heart of OCD lies a desire for control—control over one's thoughts, emotions, and surroundings. Paradoxically, the attempts to gain control through compulsive behaviors often lead to a loss of control over one's time, energy, and overall quality of life.

OCD can significantly impact daily functioning, relationships, and mental well-being. Individuals with OCD may find themselves spending hours each day performing rituals or being held captive by their obsessions, causing frustration and isolation.

## The Neurobiology of OCD

OCD has neurobiological underpinnings. Dysfunction in the brain's communication pathways, particularly involving the neurotransmitter serotonin, plays a role in the development of the disorder.

Genetic factors are also significant contributors—family history of OCD increases the likelihood of its occurrence.

## The Path to Healing

Acknowledging and addressing OCD is the first step towards healing. Professional help is crucial, as therapists trained in exposure and response prevention (ERP) therapy can guide individuals through the process of gradually facing their fears and reducing compulsive behaviors. Medications like selective serotonin reuptake inhibitors (SSRIs) can also assist in regulating neurotransmitter imbalances.

Support from loved ones is invaluable. A nonjudgmental and empathetic presence can provide solace to those struggling with the relentless loop of intrusive thoughts. Encouraging professional treatment and offering companionship can make a significant difference in the journey toward recovery.

## Breaking the Silence

Raising awareness about OCD is essential for dismantling the stigma surrounding the condition. It's crucial to recognize that individuals with OCD are not "just being picky" or "quirky." They are grappling with a complex mental health condition that deserves understanding, empathy, and support.

By fostering open conversations, dispelling misconceptions, and creating a safe space for individuals to share their experiences, we can contribute to breaking the unending loop of intrusive thoughts. With the right resources, compassionate support, and effective treatments, those affected by OCD can find solace and regain command of their lives.

## Other Relevant Conditions: A Brief Overview

Bipolar Disorder: Characterized by alternating periods of depression and mania (elevated mood, excessive energy, and impulsivity).

Schizophrenia: Involves disturbances in perception, thought, emotion, and behavior. Hallucinations, delusions, and impaired cognitive function are common.

Borderline Personality Disorder: Marked by unstable relationships, self-image, and emotions. Individuals may struggle with impulsivity and intense mood shifts.

Substance Use Disorders: Centered around the misuse of drugs or alcohol, these conditions can have profound effects on mental and physical health.

Autism Spectrum Disorder (ASD): A developmental disorder characterized by challenges in social interaction, communication, and exhibiting restricted or repetitive behaviors.

## Seeking Help and Promoting Understanding

These conditions, while diverse, share the common thread of affecting individuals' mental and emotional well-being. They are not character flaws but rather complex interactions of genetics, brain chemistry, environment, and life experiences. Understanding these conditions can foster empathy, reduce stigma, and encourage seeking appropriate professional help.

It's essential to bear in mind that mental health exists on a spectrum, and each person's experience is unique.

If you or someone you're acquainted with is grappling with any of these conditions, reaching out to a mental health professional is a vital step toward understanding, management, and recovery.

# Chapter 2

# The Science

# of

# Nutritional Psychiatry

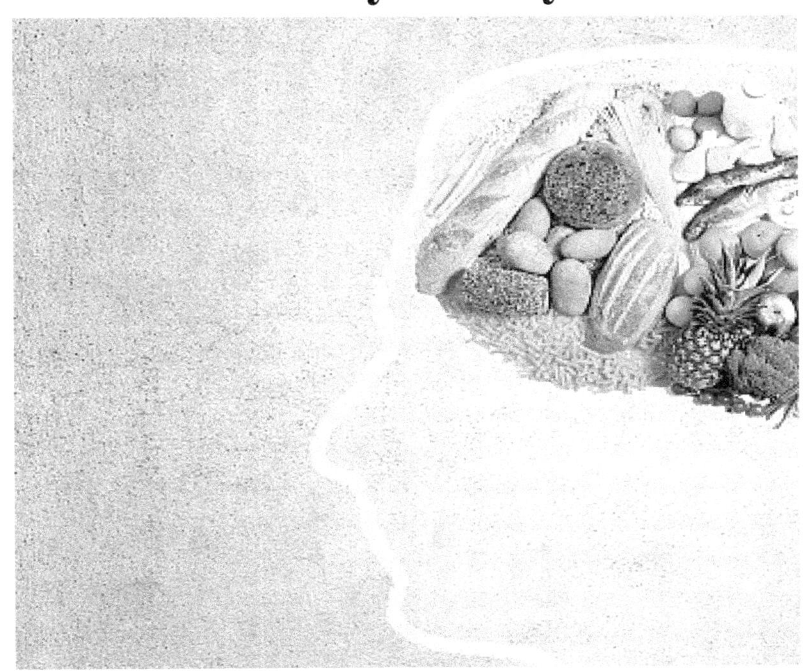

# How foods affects mental health

The age-old saying of you being what you eat feeds upon carries more truth than one may realize.

 imagine. Beyond merely satisfying hunger and providing energy, food plays a crucial role in influencing our mood and mental well-being. Recent scientific research has shed light on the intricate relationship between our dietary choices and mental health, highlighting the profound impact that certain nutrients, diets, and eating habits can change our emotional state.

The gut-brain axis is a bidirectional communication network that links the central nervous system to the enteric nervous system in the gastrointestinal tract. This connection allows the brain and gut to influence each other's function and plays a pivotal role in regulating emotions and cognitive processes. The gut is inhabited by countless microorganisms collectively referred to as the gut microbiota. Emerging evidence suggests that this complex microbial community has a significant impact on mental health.

## Nutrients and Their Impact on Mood

Certain nutrients found in foods have been shown to have a direct impact on mood regulation:Omega-3 Fatty Acids: Present in fatty fish, flaxseeds, and walnuts, omega-3 fatty acids are essential for brain health. They help maintain the structural integrity of brain cells and are linked to a reduced risk of depression and anxiety.

Vitamins and Minerals: B vitamins, particularly B6, B9 (folate), and B12, play a crucial role in neurotransmitter synthesis. Low levels of these vitamins have been associated with a higher risk of depression. Similarly, minerals like magnesium and zinc are involved in the regulation of mood-enhancing neurotransmitters.Antioxidants: Fruits and vegetables rich in antioxidants, such as vitamin C and E, help protect brain cells from oxidative stress. This protection may help reduce the risk of neurodegenerative disorders and promote overall mental well-being.

## The Impact of Diets on Mental Health

Various diets have been studied for their effects on mental health:

Mediterranean Diet: This diet, rich in fruits, vegetables, whole grains, lean protein, and healthy fats, has been linked to a lower risk of depression and cognitive decline. Its anti-inflammatory properties and abundant antioxidants contribute to its mental health benefits.

DASH Diet: The Dietary Approaches to Stop Hypertension (DASH) diet which emphasizes nutrient-rich foods and limits sodium intake, has shown promise in reducing the risk of depression and anxiety due to its positive influence on cardiovascular health.

Western Diet: On the other hand, diets high in processed foods, sugars, and unhealthy fats have been associated with a higher risk of mood disorders. The inflammatory nature of such diets can lead to oxidative stress and negatively impact brain health.

## The Role of Probiotics and Prebiotics

As previously discussed, the gut microbiota plays a substantial part in mental well-being. health. Probiotics, which are live beneficial bacteria, and prebiotics, which are non-digestible fibers that nourish these bacteria, have gained attention for their potential to improve mood and cognitive function. Probiotics may modulate the gut-brain axis, influencing neurotransmitter production and reducing inflammation, thereby promoting mental well-being.

## The Psychological Aspect of Eating

Eating isn't just a physiological process; it's also a psychological one. Binge eating, emotional eating, and restrictive eating patterns can all have negative effects on mood. Emotional eating, frequently prompted by stress or negative emotions, can lead to a vicious cycle of consuming comfort foods, which might be high in sugars and unhealthy fats. Additionally, extreme dieting or restrictive eating can deprive the body of essential nutrients, impacting brain function and emotional stability.

## Practical Tips for a Mood-Boosting Diet

Prioritize Whole Foods: Incorporate a variety of whole foods rich in nutrients and antioxidants, such as fruits, vegetables, whole grains, lean proteins, and healthy fats.

Include Omega-3s: Consume fatty fish like salmon, chia seeds, and flaxseeds to increase your intake of omega-3 fatty acids.

Moderation is Key: Enjoy sugary and processed foods in moderation, as excessive consumption can lead to blood sugar spikes and mood swings.

Dehydration affects mood and cognitive function. Adequate water throughout the day helps to reduce dehydration. Practice good eating habits, to cultivate a healthy relationship with food. Be mindful of signals of hunger and fullness.

Limit Alcohol and Caffeine: Excessive alcohol and caffeine consumption can disrupt sleep patterns and exacerbate anxiety.

The notion that food affects more than just physical health is now backed by a growing body of scientific evidence. Our food selections have a substantial impact in shaping our mood, cognitive function, and overall mental health. By adopting a balanced, nutrient-rich diet and paying attention to the gut-brain connection, we can proactively enhance our emotional well-being and promote a healthier mind. Nonetheless, it's crucial to bear in mind that even though diet is an essential factor, mental health is influenced by a multitude of factors, including genetics, environment, and social support.

## Key nutrients for brain health

The human brain, the epicenter of our cognitive abilities and emotions, requires a constant supply of essential nutrients to function optimally. Just as a well-tuned engine needs the right fuel, our brains thrive when provided with the proper nutrients. Scientific research has shown that specific vitamins, minerals, fatty acids, and antioxidants play pivotal roles in supporting brain health, enhancing cognitive function, and reducing the risk of neurodegenerative diseases. In this article, we delve into these key nutrients that contribute to the vitality of our most complex organ.

## Omega-3 Fatty Acids: The Brain's Best Friend

Omega-3 fatty acids, particularly eicosapentaenoic acid (EPA) and docosahexaenoic acid (DHA), are like superchargers for brain health. Found in abundance in fatty fish like salmon, mackerel, and sardines, these fatty acids are integral components of cell membranes in the brain and support the transmission of signals between brain cells. DHA, in particular, is highly concentrated in the brain and is crucial for cognitive function, memory, and mood regulation. Including sources of omega-3s in your diet can help reduce the risk of cognitive decline and support overall brain health.

## B Vitamins: The Cognitive Catalysts

The B vitamins are a group of water-soluble nutrients that play a vital role in brain health by contributing to the production of neurotransmitters, the brain's chemical messengers. Vitamin B6, for example, is essential for the synthesis of serotonin and dopamine, which are neurotransmitters involved in mood regulation and motivation. B vitamins, including folate (B9) and B12, also help reduce levels of homocysteine, an amino acid that, when elevated, can increase the risk of cognitive impairment and neurodegenerative diseases.

## Antioxidants:Defenders Against Oxidative Stress

Oxidative stress, caused by an imbalance between free radicals and antioxidants in the body, can lead to cell damage, inflammation, and neurodegenerative disorders. Antioxidants, such as vitamins C and E, are the body's defense against oxidative stress. Vitamin C, found in citrus fruits and berries, helps protect brain cells from damage caused by free radicals. Vitamin E, present in nuts, seeds, and leafy greens, is known for its ability to support healthy brain aging and potentially reduce the risk of Alzheimer's disease.

## Minerals for Mindfulness

Minerals like magnesium, zinc, and iron are often referred to as "mind minerals" due to their influence on cognitive function and mood regulation. Magnesium, found in leafy greens, nuts, and whole grains, facilitates approximately 600 biochemical reactions in the body, some of which are crucial for supporting brain function. health and reduce stress. Zinc is crucial for the formation of synaptic connections between brain cells, contributing to learning and memory. Iron, essential for oxygen transport in the blood, ensures that the brain receives an adequate oxygen supply, thereby maintaining optimal cognitive function.

## Choline: The Memory Molecule

Choline, often grouped with B vitamins, is a precursor to acetylcholine, a neurotransmitter that plays a vital role in memory and learning. Adequate choline intake supports the structure and function of cell membranes, aids in the transmission of nerve signals, and contributes to the development of the fetal brain during pregnancy. Eggs, lean meats, fish, and certain vegetables like broccoli are excellent sources of choline.

## Incorporating Brain-Boosting Nutrients into Your Diet

Fatty Fish: Incorporate fatty fish into your diet, aiming for at least two servings per week to boost omega-3 intake.

Leafy Greens: Consume a variety of leafy greens like spinach, kale, and Swiss chard to ensure a rich supply of antioxidants, vitamins, and minerals.

Nuts and Seeds: Snack on nuts and seeds like walnuts, flaxseeds, and almonds to increase your intake of brain-boosting omega-3s, vitamin E, and magnesium.

Colorful Fruits and Berries: Consume a rainbow of fruits and berries to provide your brain with a diverse range of antioxidants and vitamin C.

Lean Proteins: Include lean sources of protein like poultry, lean meats, eggs, and legumes to provide the building blocks for neurotransmitter synthesis.

Whole Grains: Opt for whole grains like quinoa, brown rice, and whole wheat, which provide energy and maintain a steady supply of glucose to the brain.

Our brains are remarkable organs that deserve the utmost care and attention.

A well-balanced diet rich in essential nutrients not only supports cognitive function, memory, and mood but also helps protect against the onset of neurodegenerative diseases.

By including omega-3 fatty acids, B vitamins, antioxidants, minerals, and choline into our diets, we can nourish our brains and set the stage for a vibrant and fulfilling life, where mental clarity and well-being take center stage. Remember, the power to enhance your brain health lies within the choices you make at the dining table.

# Chapter 3

# Depression-Busting Foods

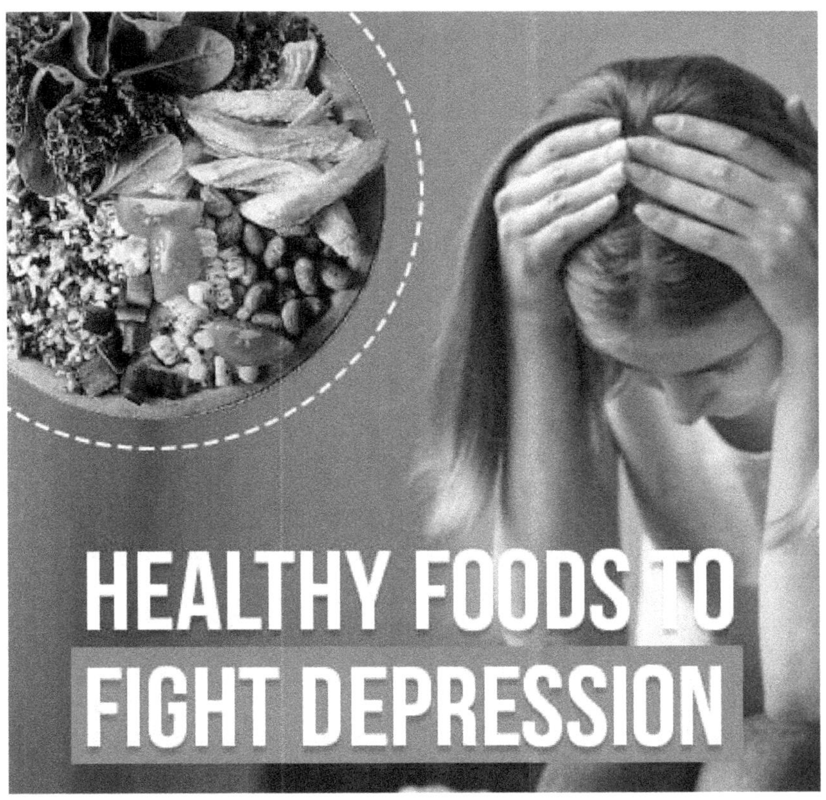

# Foods that can alleviate symptoms of depression

Depression, a prevalent mental health condition, impacts millions of individuals worldwide. While it is often treated through therapy, medication, and lifestyle changes, recent research has shown that the foods we consume can also play a significant role in alleviating the symptoms of depression. Our diets are closely linked to both our physical and mental health, and making informed dietary choices can positively impact our overall well-being. In this article, we delve into the world of nutrition and explore the foods that have the potential to alleviate symptoms of depression.

## The Gut-Brain Connection: Unraveling the Link

Before diving into specific foods, it's essential to understand the gut-brain connection and how it impacts mental health.

Gut and brain are connected through a network of nerves, hormones, and biochemical signaling systems.

This communication pathway, often referred to as the "gut-brain axis," allows for bidirectional interaction, meaning that the state of our gut health can influence our mental well-being and vice versa.

Emerging research suggests that an imbalanced gut microbiome (the collection of microorganisms living in our digestive tract) could contribute to mood disorders such as depression. Certain beneficial bacteria in the gut play a part in the production of neurotransmitters, such as serotonin, commonly known as the "feel-good" neurotransmitter. Serotonin is engaged in the regulation of mood, and its deficiency has been linked to depression. Therefore, maintaining a healthy gut microbiome through diet can indirectly impact our mental health.

## Foods That Support Mental Health

1. **Omega-3 Fatty Acids:** Found abundantly in fatty fish (such as salmon, mackerel, and sardines), flaxseeds, and walnuts, omega-3 fatty acids are noted for their anti-inflammatory attributes and potential to promote brain health. Research suggests that omega-3s may help regulate neurotransmitter function and reduce symptoms of depression.

2. **Probiotics and Fermented Foods:** Incorporating foods like yogurt, kimchi, sauerkraut, kefir, kombucha into your diet can introduce beneficial bacteria to your gut, fostering a healthier

microbiome. This, in turn, might positively influence mood regulation.

3. **Complex Carbohydrates:** Foods like whole grains, legumes, and vegetables offers a consistent source of glucose to nourish the brain. This helps stabilize blood sugar levels and prevent energy crashes that can negatively affect mood.

4. **Lean Proteins:** Protein-rich foods like lean meats, poultry, eggs, and plant-based sources (beans, lentils, tofu) contain amino acids supporting the synthesis of neurotransmitters such as dopamine and norepinephrine, which play a role in mood regulation.

5. **Leafy Greens and Colorful Vegetables:** These foods are rich in essential vitamins and minerals, including folate and magnesium. Folate is involved in serotonin production, while magnesium deficiency has been

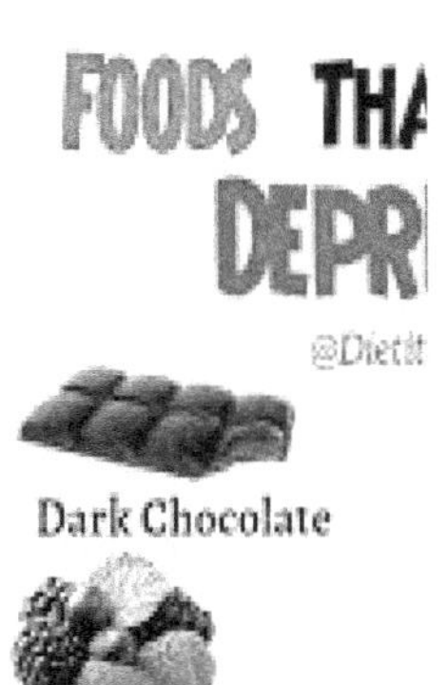

associated with a heightened risk of developing depression.

6. **Nuts and Seeds:** Almonds, cashews, and pumpkin seeds are excellent sources of magnesium, zinc, and healthy fats. These nutrients are vital for brain health and mood regulation.

7. **Dark Chocolate:** Dark chocolate contains compounds like flavonoids that have antioxidant properties. Additionally, it can trigger the release of endorphins, which contribute to feelings of pleasure and happiness.

8. **Turmeric:** The active compound in turmeric, curcumin, has anti-inflammatory and antioxidant properties. Some studies suggest that curcumin may have potential as an adjunctive treatment for depression.

## The Importance of a Balanced Diet

While these foods show promise in supporting mental health, it's important to remember that no single food can serve as a magic cure for depression. Instead, it's the overall quality and balance of your diet that truly matter. Opt for a well-rounded diet that includes a variety of nutrient-dense foods to ensure you're receiving all the necessary vitamins, minerals, and compounds that contribute to both physical and mental well-being.

Depression is a multifaceted condition shaped by a range of factors, encompassing genetics, environment, and brain chemistry. While diet alone cannot replace professional medical treatment, adopting a diet rich in omega-3 fatty acids, probiotics, whole grains, lean proteins, and colorful vegetables can contribute to improved mental well-being. The gut-brain connection highlights the profound influence our dietary choices have on mental health, emphasizing the importance of making informed decisions about the foods we consume. As research in this field continues to evolve, harnessing the power of nutrition could become an integral part of a holistic approach to managing depression and enhancing overall quality of life.

## Recipes and meal ideas

### Cooking Up Happiness: Recipes and Meal Ideas for Alleviating Depression Symptoms

In the journey towards managing and alleviating the symptoms of depression, adopting a balanced and nutritious diet can play a crucial role. The foods we consume have the potential to impact not only our physical health but also our mental well-being. Incorporating specific ingredients known to support brain health and mood regulation can contribute to a holistic approach to treating depression. In this article, we explore a variety of recipes and meal ideas created to provide sustenance for both the body and the mind.

**1. Omega-3 Rich Salmon Salad:** Omega-3 fatty acids are renowned for their positive effects on brain health. This refreshing salad combines the benefits of omega-3-rich salmon with leafy greens and a colorful assortment of vegetables.

**Ingredients:**

- Grilled or baked salmon fillet

- Mixed greens (spinach, kale, arugula)

- Cherry tomatoes

- Cucumber slices

- Red onion slices

- Avocado slices

- Walnuts or flaxseeds (for added omega-3s)

- Olive oil and lemon vinaigrette

**2. Probiotic-Packed Breakfast Bowl:** Kickstart your day with a breakfast bowl that supports gut health and provides essential nutrients for a positive mood.

**Ingredients:**

- Greek yogurt or dairy-free alternative

- Mixed berries (blueberries, strawberries, raspberries)

- Chia seeds (rich in omega-3s and fiber)

- Sliced banana

- Honey or maple syrup for sweetness

- Granola (optional)

**3. Whole Grain Buddha Bowl: A wholesome and hearty Buddha bowl incorporates complex carbohydrates, lean proteins, and a variety of colorful vegetables to fuel both body and mind.**

**Ingredients:**

- Cooked quinoa or brown rice (base)

- Grilled chicken, tofu, or chickpeas (protein)

- Steamed broccoli

- Roasted sweet potatoes

- Sliced bell peppers

- Sautéed spinach or kale

- Hummus or tahini dressing

**4. Nutrient-Rich Smoothie:** Start your day with a mood-boosting smoothie packed with vitamins, minerals, and antioxidants.

**Ingredients:**

- Spinach or kale

- Frozen mixed berries

- Banana

- Greek yogurt or nut milk

- Chia seeds or flaxseeds

- Nut butter (almond, peanut, or cashew)

- Honey or dates for sweetness

**5. Comforting Oatmeal with Nuts and Seeds:** Oats are a great source of complex carbohydrates, while nuts and seeds add healthy fats and essential nutrients.

**Ingredients:**

- Cooked rolled oats (with water or milk)

- Chopped nuts (almonds, walnuts, or pecans)

- Pumpkin seeds or sunflower seeds

- Cinnamon and nutmeg for flavor

- Sliced banana or diced apple

- Drizzle of honey or maple syrup

**6. Mood-Boosting Stir-Fry:** Stir-fry with a mix of colorful vegetables and lean protein can provide a satisfying and nutritious meal.

**Ingredients:**

- Lean protein (chicken, tofu, shrimp, or lean beef)

- Mixed stir-fry vegetables (bell peppers, broccoli, carrots, snap peas)

- Garlic and ginger for flavor

- Low-sodium soy sauce or teriyaki sauce

- Serve over brown rice or quinoa

**7. Chocolate Avocado Mousse:** Satisfy your sweet tooth with a dessert that combines the goodness of avocados and dark chocolate.

**Ingredients:**

- Ripe avocados

- Unsweetened cocoa powder

- Dark chocolate (melted)

- Honey or maple syrup for sweetness

- Vanilla extract

- Fresh berries for topping

## Conclusion: Nourishing the Mind and Body

While these recipes and meal ideas incorporate ingredients known for their potential to alleviate depression symptoms, it's important to remember that diet is just one component of a comprehensive approach to managing mental health. Professional guidance, therapy, medication (if prescribed), and a supportive environment all play crucial roles in the journey towards well-being. By embracing a balanced diet rich in nutrients that support brain health, you're taking a proactive step towards nurturing both your body and your mind.

# Chapter 4

# Anxiety-Reducing Diet

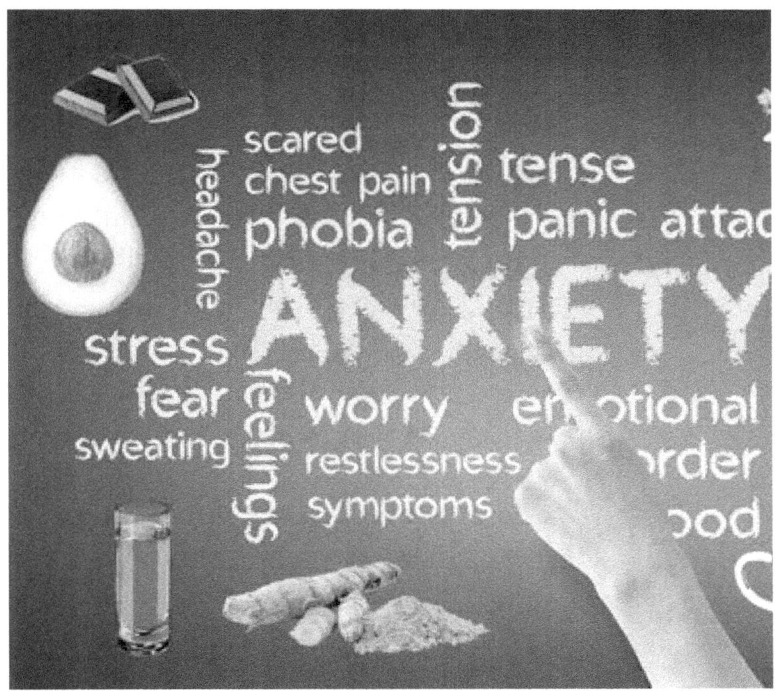

# Foods to help manage anxiety

**Cultivating Calm: Exploring the Role of Foods in Managing Anxiety**

There are conditions that can have a significant impact on a person's quality of life. Alongside traditional therapies and lifestyle adjustments, emerging research suggests that the foods we consume can play a significant role in managing anxiety symptoms.

While diet alone is not a substitute for professional treatment, making mindful dietary choices can contribute to a comprehensive approach to anxiety management. In this article, we delve into the realm of nutrition and explore the foods that have the potential to help manage anxiety.

## The Gut-Brain Connection: Unraveling the Link to Anxiety

The intricate connection between the gut and the brain, often referred to as the gut-brain axis, is becoming increasingly recognized in the world of mental health.

The gut is home to trillions of microorganisms collectively referred to as the gut microbiome. This complex ecosystem not only aids in digestion but also communicates with the brain through a network of nerves, hormones, and signaling molecules.

Recent studies have highlighted the role of the gut microbiome in influencing mood and anxiety levels. Certain beneficial bacteria in the gut play a role in producing neurotransmitters like gamma-aminobutyric acid (GABA) and serotonin, which are essential for regulating mood and reducing anxiety. Therefore, maintaining a balanced gut microbiome through diet can potentially impact anxiety symptoms.

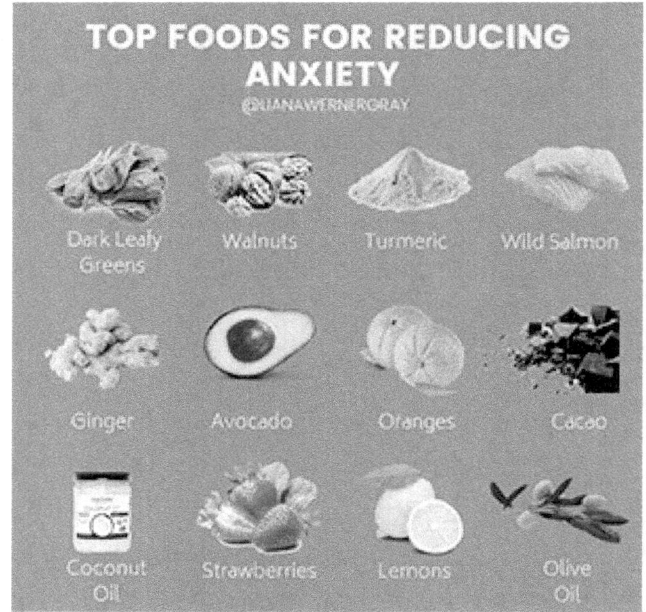


## 1. Complex Carbohydrates:

Foods such as whole grains, legumes, and vegetables offer a gradual release of glucose into the bloodstream. This helps stabilize blood sugar levels and prevents energy crashes, which can trigger or exacerbate anxiety.

2. **Leafy Greens and Colorful Vegetables:**

Nutrient-rich vegetables are packed with vitamins and minerals that support overall health, including magnesium and folate. Magnesium, in particular, has been associated with reduced anxiety levels.

3. **Fatty Fish:**Omega-3 fatty acids found in fatty fish like salmon, mackerel, and trout have anti-inflammatory properties and are believed to play a role in reducing anxiety symptoms by supporting brain health.

4. **Probiotic-RichFoods:** Incorporating fermented foods like yogurt, kefir, sauerkraut, and kimchi can introduce beneficial bacteria to the gut, potentially influencing anxiety-related neurotransmitters.

5. **Nuts and Seeds**: Walnuts, chia seeds, almonds and flax seeds are abundant

sources of nutrients. such as magnesium, zinc, and healthy fats that contribute to brain health and mood regulation.

6. **Lean Proteins:** Protein sources like lean meats, poultry, eggs, and plant-based options (beans, lentils, tofu) provide amino acids that are essential for neurotransmitter production and overall mental well-being.

7. **Dark Chocolate:** Dark chocolate contains compounds like flavonoids that have antioxidant properties. It also includes a minor quantity of caffeine, which can have mood-boosting effects.

8. **Herbal Teas:** Chamomile tea, in particular, has been linked to reduced anxiety symptoms due to its calming properties. Other herbal teas like lavender and lemon balm may also have anxiety-relieving effects.

## Balanced Eating for a Balanced Mind

While incorporating these anxiety-friendly foods into your diet, it's crucial to focus on balance and moderation. Overindulgence or restriction of any specific food group can potentially have negative effects on overall well-being. Moreover, staying hydrated by drinking sufficient water throughout the day is essential for maintaining cognitive function and managing anxiety.

## Conclusion: A Holistic Approach to Anxiety Management

Anxiety management is a multifaceted journey that involves various aspects of life, including professional guidance, therapy, physical activity, and diet. While certain foods have the potential to support anxiety management by influencing brain chemistry and gut health, they should be seen as part of a broader strategy rather than a standalone solution. Individual responses to foods can vary, so paying attention to how your body and mind react to different dietary choices is crucial. By cultivating a diet that prioritizes nutrient-rich, anxiety-friendly foods, you can contribute to a holistic approach to managing anxiety and nurturing your mental well-being.

# Meal plans for anxiety

**Nurturing Tranquility: Crafting Meal Plans for Anxiety Relief**

Anxiety, a common mental health concern, affects millions of individuals around the world. Alongside therapy, lifestyle changes, and professional treatment, the foods we consume can have a significant impact on anxiety management. Developing a thoughtfully designed meal plan can provide the body with essential nutrients that support mental well-being. In this article, we'll explore the concept of creating meal plans tailored to alleviating anxiety symptoms.

# The Nutritional Approach to Anxiety Management

Anxiety can originate from a range of factors, including genetics, environment, and brain chemistry. While diet alone cannot replace professional treatment, adopting a diet rich in specific nutrients can contribute to a holistic approach to managing anxiety. Nutrients like omega-3 fatty acids, magnesium, B vitamins, and antioxidants are known to play a role in supporting brain health and reducing anxiety.

## Creating a Balanced Meal Plan

Building a meal plan that addresses anxiety involves selecting foods that nourish both the body and the mind. Here's an overview of what constitutes a well-balanced meal plan for anxiety relief might look like:

**Breakfast:** Begin the day with a breakfast that provides sustained energy and essential nutrients.

- **Option 1:** Greek yogurt parfait with mixed berries, chia seeds, and a drizzle of honey. Pair with whole-grain toast or a small serving of oatmeal.

- **Option 2:** Scrambled eggs with spinach, tomatoes, and a sprinkle of feta cheese. Serve with whole-grain toast and a side of avocado.

**Mid-Morning Snack:** Opt for a snack that maintains energy levels and supports focus.

- **Option 1:** A small handful of mixed nuts (almonds, walnuts) and a piece of fruit.

- **Option 2:** Carrot and cucumber sticks with hummus for dipping.

**Lunch:** Choose a lunch that includes lean protein, complex carbohydrates, and plenty of vegetables.

- **Option 1:** Grilled chicken salad with mixed greens, quinoa, cherry tomatoes, cucumber slices, and a light vinaigrette.

- **Option 2:** Veggie wrap with hummus, roasted red peppers, spinach, shredded carrots, and whole-grain tortilla.

**Afternoon Snack:** Select a snack that provides sustained energy and contains anxiety-supportive nutrients.

- **Option 1:** Greek yogurt with a sprinkle of nuts, seeds, and a dash of cinnamon.

- **Option 2:** Apple slices with almond butter.

**Dinner:** Opt for a well-balanced dinner that combines lean protein, whole grains, and a variety of vegetables.

- **Option 1:** Baked salmon with quinoa and a side of steamed broccoli, asparagus, and bell peppers.

- **Option 2:** Lentil soup with whole-grain bread and a side salad of mixed greens, avocado, and sunflower seeds.

**Evening Snack:** Choose a light, soothing snack that encourages relaxation.

- **Option 1:** Herbal tea (chamomile, lavender) with a small piece of dark chocolate.

- **Option 2:** Sliced banana with a drizzle of honey and a sprinkle of nuts or seeds.

Hydration: Maintain proper hydration throughout the day by consuming water, herbal teas, and infusions.

## Final Thoughts

Crafting a meal plan for anxiety management involves embracing a wide variety of nutrient-dense foods that can positively impact brain health and mood regulation. Nonetheless, individual reactions to foods can differ, so it's crucial to pay attention to your body and adapt based on your distinct needs and preferences.

A holistic approach to anxiety management includes professional guidance, therapy, lifestyle adjustments, and a supportive environment.

By thoughtfully planning meals that prioritize anxiety-supportive nutrients, you're taking a proactive step toward nurturing your mental well-being.

# Chapter 5

# PTSD and Nutrition

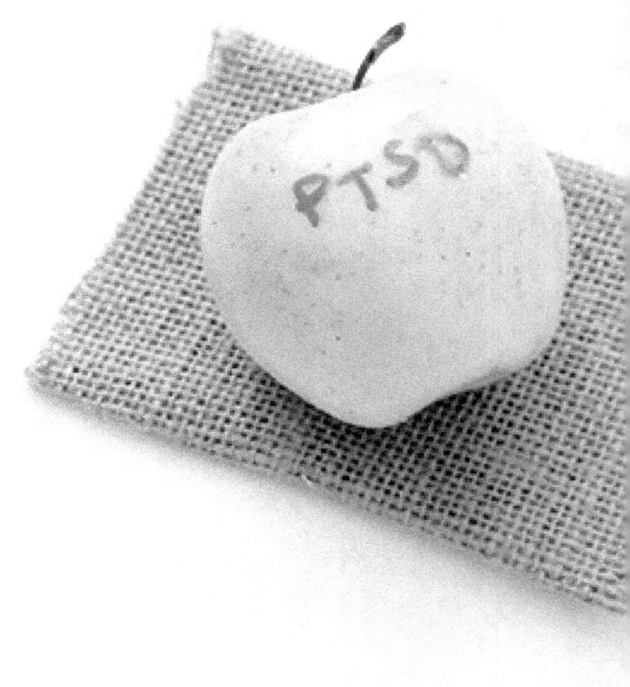

# Nutritional strategies for coping with PTSD

**Empowering Recovery: Nutritional Strategies for Coping with PTSD**

Post-Traumatic Stress Disorder (PTSD) is a complex and often debilitating mental health condition that can result from exposure to traumatic events. While professional treatment, therapy, and support are essential components of managing PTSD, emerging research suggests that nutrition can play a role in supporting the recovery process. Nutritional strategies can contribute to overall well-being, alleviate symptoms, and enhance resilience. In this comprehensive article, we explore the connection between nutrition and PTSD, and delve into effective nutritional strategies for coping with the condition.

# The Nutrition-Mental Health Connection

The intricate relationship between nutrition and mental health is gaining recognition as research uncovers the impact of diet on brain function and mood regulation.

The brain necessitates a well-rounded intake of nutrients to operate efficiently, and deficiencies can affect neurotransmitter production, hormone regulation, and overall mental well-being.

For individuals coping with PTSD, targeted nutritional strategies can complement therapeutic interventions and contribute to a more holistic approach to recovery.

## Nutritional Strategies for Coping with PTSD:

1. **Balanced Macronutrient Intake:** A well-rounded diet that includes a balance of carbohydrates, proteins, and healthy fats supports stable blood sugar

levels, which can have a positive impact on mood stability. Avoiding extreme diets and prioritizing whole foods can provide sustained energy and prevent energy crashes that may exacerbate PTSD symptoms.

2. **Omega-3 Fatty Acids:** Foods rich in omega-3 fatty acids, such as fatty fish (salmon, mackerel), flaxseeds, and walnuts, have anti-inflammatory properties and are associated with improved brain health. Omega-3s can potentially reduce symptoms of anxiety and depression often associated with PTSD.

3. **B Vitamins:** B vitamins, particularly B6, B9 (folate), and B12, play a role in neurotransmitter production and are essential for brain health. Leafy greens, legumes, fortified cereals, lean meats, and dairy products are good sources of these vitamins.

4. **Antioxidant-Rich Foods:** Incorporating a variety of colorful fruits and vegetables provides essential antioxidants that combat oxidative stress and inflammation. Citrus fruits, dark leafy greens, berries, and bell peppers are excellent sources of essential nutrients.

5. **Probiotics and Gut Health:** Emerging research suggests a strong connection between the gut microbiome and mental health. Consuming probiotic-rich foods (yogurt, kefir, fermented vegetables) and high-fiber foods supports gut health, potentially influencing mood regulation.

6. **Complex Carbohydrates:** Whole grains like brown rice, quinoa, and oats provide a steady release of glucose, promoting stable energy levels and preventing blood sugar fluctuations that can impact mood.

7. **Lean Proteins:** Incorporate lean protein sources like poultry, fish, beans, and tofu. Proteins contain amino acids necessary for neurotransmitter production and can contribute to improved mood.

8. **Hydration:** Staying hydrated is crucial for cognitive function and overall well-being. Opt for water, herbal teas, and natural juices to maintain adequate hydration.

9. **Mindful Eating Practices:** Practicing mindful eating can help create a positive relationship with food. Always give adequate attention to the way you eat.

## Individualized Approach and Professional Guidance

It's crucial to acknowledge that individual reactions to particular foods can differ. Seeking guidance from a healthcare expert, such as a registered dietitian or nutritionist, can help tailor nutritional strategies to an individual's needs and circumstances.

Conclusion: Integrating Nutrition into PTSD Recovery

While nutritional strategies are not a standalone solution for coping with PTSD, they can complement therapeutic interventions and contribute to a more comprehensive approach to recovery. The connection between nutrition and mental health is complex, and making informed dietary choices can have a positive impact on mood, energy levels, and overall well-being. By embracing a balanced and nutrient-rich diet, individuals with PTSD can empower themselves on their journey towards healing and resilience.

# Stories of individuals who have benefited from dietary changes

## From Trauma to Triumph: Inspiring Stories of PTSD Recovery Through Dietary Changes

Post-Traumatic Stress Disorder (PTSD) can cast a heavy shadow over an individual's life, which can be significantly influenced, affecting their mental, emotional, and physical well-being. While traditional therapies and medical interventions are vital in the journey to recovery, dietary changes have shown remarkable promise in contributing to the alleviation of PTSD symptoms. In this article, we share inspiring stories of individuals who have triumphed over their traumatic experiences and found relief from PTSD through intentional dietary changes.

*Sarah's Journey to Healing Through Nutrition*

Sarah, a survivor of a car accident that left her with both physical and emotional scars, struggled with nightmares, anxiety, and mood swings for years after the incident. Feeling frustrated by the limitations that PTSD imposed on her life, she decided to explore alternative approaches to healing. After extensive research and consulting with healthcare professionals, Sarah overhauled her diet to include foods rich in omega-3 fatty acids, antioxidants, and complex carbohydrates.

She incorporated fatty fish like salmon and mackerel into her meals, focusing on their omega-3 content known for supporting brain health. She also added a variety of colorful fruits and vegetables to her diet to boost her intake of antioxidants, which combat oxidative stress linked to anxiety and depression. By adopting whole grains and lean proteins, Sarah ensured that her blood sugar levels remained stable, leading to improved mood stability.

Over time, Sarah noticed a significant reduction in her anxiety levels, fewer nightmares, and an overall sense of well-being. While dietary changes weren't a standalone solution, they became a crucial part of her holistic approach to recovery. Sarah's journey highlights the importance of understanding the connection between nutrition and mental health and tailoring dietary choices to individual needs.

*John's Path to Freedom from PTSD Symptoms*

John, a military veteran, faced PTSD symptoms that included intrusive thoughts, hypervigilance, and irritability stemming from his combat experiences. Seeking ways to regain control over his life, John delved into research about the impact of diet on mental health. He was particularly intrigued by studies showcasing the potential benefits of probiotics in alleviating anxiety and depression.

John began consuming fermented foods like yogurt, kefir, and sauerkraut, which introduced beneficial bacteria to his gut. As he continued to prioritize gut health through his dietary choices, he noticed subtle shifts in his mood and overall outlook. With the guidance of a mental health professional, he combined dietary changes with therapy, gradually experiencing a reduction in the intensity and frequency of his PTSD symptoms.

The progress John made in managing his PTSD was a testament to the synergy between evidence-based therapies and nutritional strategies. His story underscores the importance of taking a holistic approach to recovery and the potential of dietary changes to complement traditional interventions.

*Rachel's Renewed Hope Through Mindful Eating*

Rachel, a survivor of domestic violence, faced severe anxiety, flashbacks, and emotional numbness due to her traumatic experiences. In her journey towards healing, she discovered the power of mindful eating. Rachel practiced intuitive eating, paying close attention to her body's hunger and fullness cues while savoring the flavors of each meal.

By nurturing a healthy relationship with food, Rachel found that her emotional eating tendencies diminished. She naturally gravitated towards whole, nutrient-dense foods that supported her overall well-being. Over time, her improved relationship with food coincided with reduced anxiety levels and fewer intrusive thoughts.

Rachel's experience showcases the importance of considering the emotional aspect of eating when addressing PTSD symptoms. By embracing mindful eating, individuals like Rachel can find solace and renewed hope in their recovery journey.

Conclusion: A Path to Empowerment

The stories of Sarah, John, and Rachel illustrate the potential of dietary changes in contributing to the recovery from PTSD. While their journeys were uniquely tailored to their needs, the common thread is the empowerment that came from taking control of their well-being. As these individuals discovered, dietary changes can complement traditional therapies, fostering a comprehensive approach to managing PTSD symptoms. The path to recovery may be challenging, but these stories stand as beacons of hope for those seeking relief from the burdens of trauma.

# Chapter 6

# ADHD and Dietary Interventions

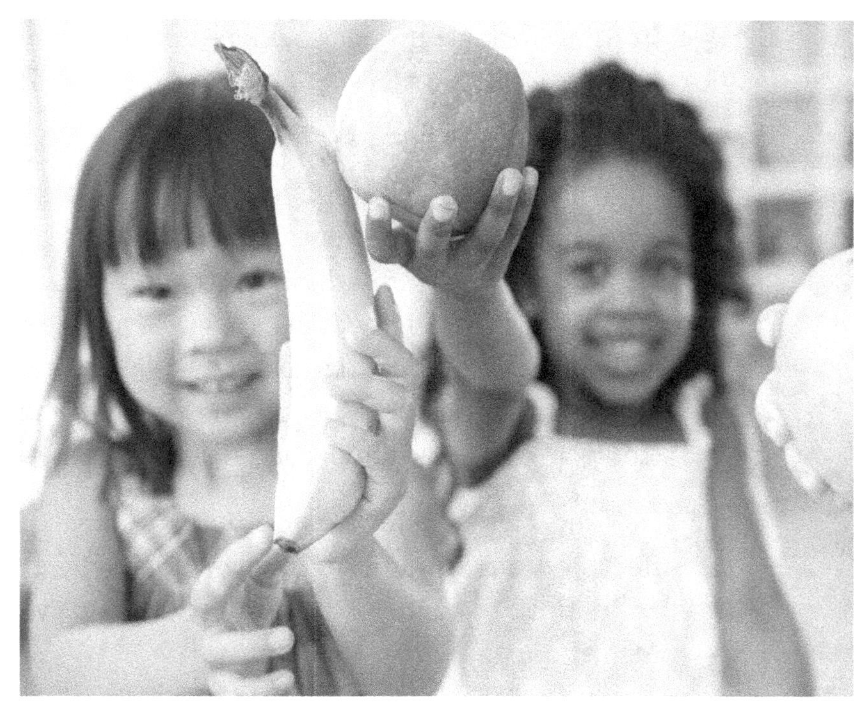

# How diet can impact attention and hyperactivity

Mindful Nutrition: Exploring the Intricate Link Between Diet and Attention-Hyperactivity

Attention and hyperactivity are essential components of cognitive function, particularly in children and individuals with conditions like Attention-Deficit/Hyperactivity Disorder (ADHD). Emerging research suggests that diet plays a significant role in influencing attention, focus, and hyperactivity levels.

The foods we consume contain nutrients that affect brain function, neurotransmitter production, and overall cognitive performance.

In this article, we delve into the complex relationship between diet and attention-hyperactivity, exploring how dietary choices can impact cognitive functioning.

## The Role of Nutrients in Brain Function

The brain is a highly energy-demanding organ that relies on a steady supply of nutrients to function optimally. Nutrients like vitamins, minerals, amino acids, and fatty acids play vital roles in neurotransmitter synthesis, nerve communication, and cognitive processes. Therefore, the quality of our diet directly influences how our brain functions, including our ability to focus and control hyperactivity.

Dietary Factors Affecting Attention and Hyperactivity:

1. **Omega-3 Fatty Acids:** These essential fats, found in fatty fish (salmon, mackerel), flaxseeds, walnuts, and chia seeds, are crucial for brain health. Omega-3s are known to support neurotransmitter function, reduce inflammation, and enhance cognitive performance. Research suggests that omega-3 supplementation may have a positive impact on attention and hyperactivity in children with ADHD.

2. **Protein and Amino Acids:** Protein-rich foods like lean meats, poultry, fish, beans, and legumes supply the essential amino acids required for neurotransmitter production. Amino acids such as tryptophan and tyrosine are precursors to serotonin and dopamine, which influence mood, focus, and attention.

3. **Complex Carbohydrates:** Foods like whole grains, fruits, and vegetables offer a gradual release of glucose into the bloodstream, supplying the brain with a consistent source of energy. This helps maintain stable energy levels, reducing fluctuations that can affect attention and hyperactivity.

4. **Vitamins and Minerals:** Nutrients like B vitamins, zinc, iron, and magnesium are essential for cognitive function. Deficiencies in these nutrients have been associated with poor attention,

cognitive impairments, and behavioral issues.

5. **Sugars and Processed Foods:** High sugar consumption and processed foods with artificial additives can lead to energy spikes followed by crashes, impacting attention and contributing to hyperactivity. A diet high in refined sugars has been linked to increased symptoms of ADHD in some studies.

6. **Hydration:** Dehydration can negatively affect cognitive performance, leading to difficulty concentrating and irritability. Staying adequately hydrated throughout the day is crucial for maintaining attention.

Mindful Eating for Improved Attention-Hyperactivity Management:

1. **Balanced Meals:** Prioritize meals that include a balance of macronutrients – lean proteins, complex carbohydrates,

and healthy fats. A balanced diet supports stable energy levels and cognitive function.

2. **Consistent Meals and Snacks:** Consuming regular meals and snacks throughout the day prevents blood sugar fluctuations, ensuring a steady supply of energy for the brain.

3. **Incorporate Omega-3s:** Include sources of omega-3 fatty acids in your diet to support brain health. Consider fatty fish, flaxseeds, chia seeds, and walnuts.

4. **Colorful Fruits and Vegetables:** Consume a variety of colorful fruits and vegetables to provide essential vitamins, minerals, and antioxidants for cognitive support.

5. **Limit Sugar and Processed Foods:** Reduce the consumption of sugary snacks, beverages, and heavily

processed foods to prevent energy crashes and support stable attention.

Conclusion: A Nutrient-Rich Path to Improved Cognitive Function

While diet alone cannot replace professional treatment for conditions like ADHD, the evidence suggests that mindful nutrition can significantly impact attention and hyperactivity. By making informed dietary choices that prioritize nutrient-dense foods, individuals can support their cognitive function, enhance focus, and manage hyperactivity more effectively. A holistic approach to cognitive well-being considers diet as a foundational pillar, fostering optimal brain health and cognitive performance.

# Tips for parents and children

Navigating ADHD: Expert Dietary Tips for Parents and Children

Attention-Deficit/Hyperactivity Disorder (ADHD) is a neurodevelopmental condition that impacts an individual's capacity to concentrate, regulate impulses, and handle hyperactivity. While ADHD is commonly managed through a combination of therapies, medications, and support, emerging research suggests that dietary choices can play a role in alleviating symptoms and improving overall well-being. For parents and caregivers of children with ADHD, understanding the impact of diet and implementing appropriate dietary strategies can be a valuable addition to their approach. In this comprehensive article, we provide expert dietary tips tailored for parents and children dealing with ADHD.

The Diet-ADHD Connection: Unveiling the Influence

The relationship between diet and ADHD is complex, and while diet cannot be seen as a standalone treatment, it can contribute to symptom management and improved cognitive function. Certain nutrients impact brain health, neurotransmitter production, and cognitive processes, which are essential for individuals with ADHD. Additionally, stabilizing blood sugar levels, promoting gut health, and reducing inflammation can indirectly affect attention and hyperactivity.

Dietary Tips for Parents:

1. **Balanced and Regular Meals:** Prioritize balanced meals that include lean proteins, complex carbohydrates, and healthy fats. Regular meals and snacks throughout the day can prevent blood sugar fluctuations that might worsen ADHD symptoms.

2. **Omega-3 Fatty Acids:** Incorporate fatty fish (salmon, mackerel), flaxseeds, walnuts, and chia seeds into your child's

diet. Omega-3s support brain health and cognitive function, potentially alleviating ADHD symptoms.

3. **Limit Processed Foods:** Reduce the consumption of sugary snacks, artificial additives, and heavily processed foods. These can lead to energy crashes and negatively impact focus and behavior.

4. **High-fiber Foods:** like whole grains, fruits, and vegetables. Fiber promotes stable blood sugar levels and supports gut health.

5. **Protein-Rich Snacks:** Offer protein-rich snacks such as yogurt, cheese, nuts, and lean meats. Protein helps stabilize energy levels and enhances neurotransmitter production.

6. **Hydration:** helps children stay adequately hydrated throughout the day. Dehydration can affect cognitive function and behavior.

Dietary Tips for Children with ADHD:

1. **Mindful Eating:** Encourage your child to eat mindfully, focusing on each bite and eating slowly. This practice can aid in enhancing digestion and reducing the likelihood of overeating.

2. **Colorful Fruits and Vegetables:** Incorporate a variety of colorful fruits and vegetables into their meals. These provide essential vitamins, minerals, and antioxidants that support brain health.

3. **Reduce Sugary Beverages:** Cut back on sugary drinks and choose water, herbal teas, and natural juices. Avoiding excessive sugar can prevent energy crashes and mood swings.

4. **Homemade Snacks:** Prepare homemade snacks that combine protein and complex carbohydrates. Examples

include apple slices with peanut butter or whole-grain crackers with cheese.

5. **Cook Together:** Engage your child in the process of meal planning and cooking. This can encourage a positive relationship with food and a willingness to try new, nutrient-rich options.

Consulting a Professional:

It's important to consult a healthcare professional before making significant dietary changes, especially for children with ADHD. A registered dietitian or pediatrician can provide guidance tailored to your child's specific needs and preferences.

Conclusion: A Holistic Approach to ADHD Management

Dietary strategies for parents and children dealing with ADHD can serve as complementary tools to traditional treatments. While there is no one-size-fits-all approach, the emphasis on nutrient-rich, balanced meals can positively impact cognitive function, attention, and behavior. Combining dietary choices with therapies, medications (if prescribed), and a supportive environment can create a comprehensive approach to managing ADHD symptoms. Remember that patience, understanding, and collaboration with healthcare professionals are key to achieving the best outcomes for children with ADHD.

# Chapter 7

# OCD and Nutritional Support

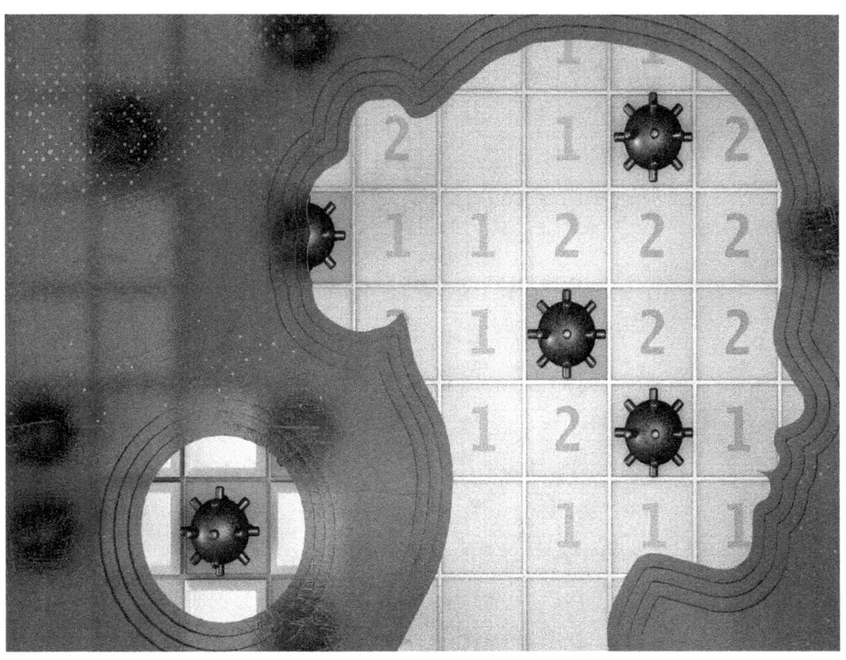

# Foods that may ease symptoms of OCD

Obsessive-Compulsive Disorder (OCD) is a mental health disorder distinguished by intrusive thoughts (obsessions) and repetitive behaviors (compulsions). While it's primarily treated through therapy, medication, and lifestyle changes, emerging research suggests that certain dietary choices can play a role in managing OCD symptoms. The foods we consume can influence brain health, neurotransmitter production, and overall well-being. In this article, we delve into the potential connection between diet and OCD, exploring foods that might alleviate symptoms and promote a sense of calm.

The Gut-Brain Axis: Unveiling the Connection

The gut-brain axis, a complex communication network between the gut and the brain, has garnered increasing attention in the field of mental health. The gut microbiome, the assemblage of microorganisms residing in our digestive system, plays a significant role in this connection. Research indicates that an imbalanced gut microbiome may contribute to mental health conditions, including OCD. Certain beneficial bacteria in the gut are involved in producing neurotransmitters like serotonin, which plays a role in mood regulation and anxiety reduction.

Foods That May Alleviate OCD Symptoms:

1. **Omega-3 Fatty Acids:** Fatty fish (salmon, mackerel, sardines), flaxseeds, chia seeds, and walnuts are rich in omega-3 fatty acids. These fats have anti-inflammatory properties and support brain health. Omega-3s might contribute to reducing symptoms of

anxiety and depression often associated with OCD.

2. **Probiotic-Rich Foods**: Adding fermented foods such as yogurt, kefir, sauerkraut, and kimchi can introduce beneficial bacteria to the gut. A healthy gut microbiome may indirectly influence mood and anxiety levels.

3. **Carbohydrates** Foods: like whole grains, legumes, and vegetables offer a consistent source of glucose to support brain function. This prevents energy crashes and helps stabilize mood.

4. **Lean Proteins:** Including lean protein sources like poultry, fish, beans, and lentils provides amino acids necessary for neurotransmitter production. These amino acids play a role in mood regulation and overall mental well-being.

5. **Antioxidant-Rich Foods:** Berries, dark leafy greens, nuts, and seeds are rich in antioxidants that combat oxidative stress and inflammation. Reducing oxidative stress may contribute to reducing anxiety symptoms.

6. **Dark Chocolate:** Dark chocolate contains compounds like flavonoids that have antioxidant properties. Additionally, it can trigger the release of endorphins, which contribute to feelings of pleasure and happiness.

7. **Magnesium-Rich Foods:** Leafy greens, nuts, seeds, and whole grains provide magnesium, a mineral that is involved in neurotransmitter function and can have a calming effect on the nervous system.

8. **Herbal Teas:** Chamomile tea and lemon balm tea are known for their calming properties. These herbal infusions can

promote relaxation and alleviate symptoms of anxiety.

A Holistic Approach to Wellness:

While dietary choices can play a role in managing OCD symptoms, they are just one aspect of a comprehensive approach to mental health. Seeking professional guidance, engaging in therapy, practicing stress-reduction techniques, and maintaining a supportive environment are equally important components of well-rounded OCD management.

Conclusion: Nurturing Mental Well-being Through Nutrition

The journey to managing OCD involves multiple elements, with diet serving as a potential complement to traditional therapies. While no single food can cure OCD, a diet rich in nutrients that support brain health, reduce inflammation, and promote overall well-being may contribute to alleviating symptoms and enhancing the quality of life for individuals with OCD. By embracing a balanced and nutrient-dense diet, individuals can take a proactive step toward nurturing their mental well-being and fostering a sense of calm amidst the challenges of OCD.

## Personal anecdotes and success stories

Personal Journeys of Triumph: Inspiring Anecdotes and Success Stories from the Battle Against OCD

Obsessive-Compulsive Disorder (OCD) can cast a shadow over every aspect of life, but for those who have faced its challenges head-on, the journey toward recovery serves as a testament to the remarkable resilience and unwavering determination of the human spirit. Personal anecdotes and success stories from individuals who have battled OCD shed light on the strength it takes to confront this mental health condition and the hope that recovery is possible. In this article, we explore some inspiring stories of individuals who have triumphed over their OCD and offer hope to others on a similar path.

*Sarah's Story: A Journey to Self-Discovery*

Sarah's life was once dictated by her obsessions and compulsions. Counting, checking, and cleaning rituals consumed her days, leaving her feeling trapped and isolated. However, her turning point came when she decided to confront her fears head-on through Exposure and Response Prevention (ERP) therapy. With the support of her therapist, she gradually faced her triggers, allowing the anxiety to peak without engaging in compulsions. Over time, her anxiety diminished, and she regained control over her life.

Sarah's story highlights the importance of seeking professional help and the courage it takes to face the discomfort of ERP therapy. Her journey from a a place of darkness to a state of empowerment demonstrates a profound transformation power of confronting OCD headfirst.



Jake's struggle with OCD centered around intrusive thoughts that would terrify him. His daily life was a constant battle against these unwelcome mental images. His turning point came when he joined a support group for individuals with OCD. Sharing his experiences with others who understood his struggles provided a sense of relief and community. Jake combined therapy with mindfulness practices and exercise, which helped him gain control over his thoughts and reduce his anxiety.

Jake's story emphasizes the significance of community support and holistic approaches to managing OCD. His journey from fear and isolation to empowerment and self-acceptance showcases the possibilities that open up when individuals find the right combination of strategies that work for them.



Lily's OCD revolved around the need for symmetry and perfection in her daily life. Every activity, from arranging objects to completing tasks, had to adhere to her strict mental rules. But Lily's breakthrough came when she realized that her pursuit of perfection was hindering her ability to enjoy life. With therapy, she learned to challenge her compulsions and accept the discomfort that came with it. Through practicing self-compassion and reframing her thoughts, Lily started to embrace imperfections and let go of the need for rigid control.

Lily's story showcases the importance of self-compassion and acceptance in the journey to managing OCD. Her transformation from a life bound by rigid rules to a life full of spontaneity and joy illustrates the power of shifting perspectives.

Conclusion: Stories of Strength and Hope

Personal anecdotes and success stories from individuals who have faced and triumphed over OCD serve as beacons of hope for others on a similar journey. These stories remind us that while the path to recovery may be challenging, it is possible to overcome the grip of OCD and regain control over one's life. The shared themes of seeking help, confronting fears, finding support, and embracing self-compassion are a testament to the resilience of the human spirit. As these stories show, there is light at the end of the tunnel for those navigating the labyrinth of OCD, and each step toward recovery is a victory worth celebrating.

# Chapter 8

# Other Mental Health Condition

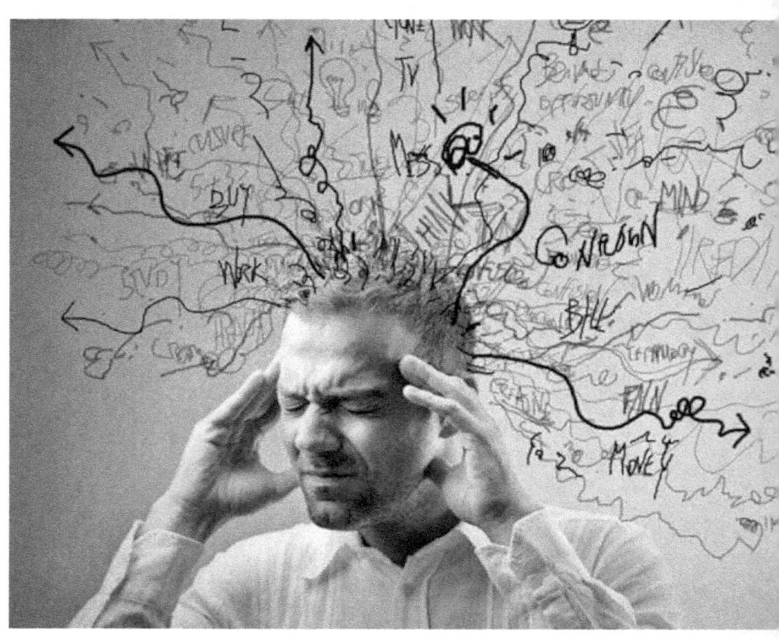

# Exploring how nutrition can aid in managing other conditions like bipolar disorder, schizophrenia, and more

## Bipolar Disorder

Bipolar disorder, also known as manic-depressive illness, is a complex and often debilitating mental health condition characterized by extreme mood swings. People with bipolar disorder experience episodes of mania (elevated mood, increased energy) and depression (low mood, lack of energy), which can severely disrupt their daily lives. While medication and therapy are the primary treatments for bipolar disorder, emerging research suggests that nutrition may also play a significant role in managing and mitigating the symptoms of this disorder.

In this article, we will delve into the relationship between nutrition and bipolar disorder and explore how dietary choices can help individuals better manage their condition.

The Bipolar-Nutrition Connection

1.  Omega-3 Fatty Acids:

Omega-3 fatty acids, primarily found in fatty fish like salmon, mackerel, and trout, have long been touted for their various health benefits, including their potential role in managing bipolar disorder. Research has shown that omega-3s can help reduce the severity and frequency of mood swings in individuals with bipolar disorder. These essential fatty acids have anti-inflammatory properties and are thought to help regulate brain function, which may contribute to mood stabilization.

2.  Micronutrients:

Micronutrients, which encompass vitamins and minerals, are fundamental for maintaining overall health and well-being. Several studies have explored the link between micronutrient deficiencies and bipolar disorder. Deficiencies in certain vitamins and minerals, such as vitamin D, vitamin B12, and magnesium, have been associated with an increased risk of mood instability and depressive symptoms. Ensuring an adequate intake of these nutrients through diet or supplementation may help manage bipolar symptoms.

3. Gut-Brain Connection:

The gut-brain connection is an emerging field of research that explores the intricate relationship between the digestive system and mental health. The gut microbiome, a community of trillions of microorganisms residing in the digestive tract plays a pivotal role in facilitating this connection. Emerging evidence suggests that an imbalanced gut microbiome may contribute to mood disorders, including bipolar disorder. Diet is a major influencer of gut microbiota composition, so adopting a diet rich in fiber, fermented foods, and prebiotics can potentially support a healthier gut-brain axis.

4. Blood Sugar Regulation:

Balancing blood sugar levels is essential for overall health, and it may be particularly relevant for individuals with bipolar disorder. Fluctuations in blood sugar levels can impact mood stability and energy levels. A diet that focuses on complex carbohydrates, high-fiber foods, and balanced meals can help stabilize blood sugar levels and potentially reduce mood swings.

5. Amino Acids:

Specific amino acids, including tryptophan and tyrosine, serve as precursors to neurotransmitters like serotonin and dopamine, which hold significant importance in mood regulation. Incorporating foods rich in these amino acids, such as turkey (tryptophan) and lean meats (tyrosine), may contribute to more stable moods.

6. Caffeine and Alcohol:

Caffeine and alcohol are known to affect mood and can exacerbate the symptoms of bipolar disorder. Caffeine can disrupt sleep patterns and trigger manic episodes, while alcohol is a depressant that can worsen depressive symptoms. Reducing or eliminating the consumption of these substances can have a positive impact on mood stability.

Challenges in Dietary Management of Bipolar Disorder

While nutrition can indeed play a role in managing bipolar disorder, it is important to acknowledge the challenges individuals with this condition may face when trying to make dietary changes. Some of these challenges include:

1. Medication Interactions: Many individuals with bipolar disorder are prescribed medication to manage their symptoms. Some dietary choices and supplements may interact with these medications, making it crucial for individuals to seek guidance from their healthcare providers before making significant dietary changes.

2. Emotional Eating: Most times the way we eat addresses the emotional aspects of nutrition in the body and that can be challenging to our health.

3. Nutritional Deficiencies: Bipolar disorder itself can impact appetite and dietary choices, potentially leading to nutritional deficiencies. Working with a healthcare team to monitor and address these deficiencies is crucial.

4. Individual Variability: Nutrition is not a one-size-fits-all solution. What works for one individual dealing with bipolar

disorder may not be effective for someone else. It's essential for individuals to work with healthcare professionals to develop personalized dietary strategies.

Conclusion

While nutrition is not a standalone treatment for bipolar disorder, it can be a valuable complementary approach to help manage and mitigate the symptoms of this complex condition. A well-rounded diet abundant in omega-3 fatty acids, micronutrients, and foods that support gut health, along with attention to blood sugar regulation and the avoidance of mood-altering substances, can contribute to more stable moods and improved overall well-being for individuals with bipolar disorder. Nevertheless, it is crucial for individuals to work closely with their healthcare providers to tailor their dietary strategies to their unique needs and circumstances as part of a comprehensive treatment plan.



Breakfast:

Omega-3 Smoothie: Blend spinach, banana, frozen berries, chia seeds (for omega-3s), and a splash of almond milk for a nutritious and mood-stabilizing start to your day.

Mid-Morning Snack:

Greek Yogurt Parfait: Top Greek yogurt with fresh berries and a drizzle of honey for a protein-packed and satisfying snack.

Lunch:

Salmon Salad: Grill or bake salmon and serve it over a bed of mixed greens, cherry tomatoes, cucumber, and avocado. Add a lemon vinaigrette drizzle for an extra burst of flavor.

Afternoon Snack:

Carrot Sticks with Hummus: Carrots are rich in fiber, and hummus provides protein and healthy fats, making this a balanced and convenient snack.

Dinner:

Quinoa-Stuffed Bell Peppers: Combine cooked quinoa with black beans, diced tomatoes, corn, and spices. Fill the mixture into bell peppers and bake until they become tender.

Dessert (if desired):

Dark Chocolate: A small piece of dark chocolate can satisfy sweet cravings without causing blood sugar spikes.

Recipes for Bipolar-Friendly Meals

**Omega-3 Salmon Fillet:**

Ingredients:

2 salmon fillets

2 tablespoons olive oil

1 lemon, thinly sliced

Salt and pepper to taste

Instructions:

Preheat your oven to 375°F (190°C).

Here are the steps:

1. Lay the salmon filets on a baking paper with parchment paper.
2. Pour little olive oil over the salmon and season with salt and pepper.

3. Put lemon slices on top of each filet.

This will help create a delicious lemon-infused baked salmon dish.

4.  Allow to bake for 15-20 minutes .

## Mood-Stabilizing Omega-3 Smoothie:

Ingredients:

1 cup fresh spinach leaves

1 banana

1/2 cup frozen berries (e.g., blueberries or strawberries)

1 tablespoon chia seeds

1 cup unsweetened almond milk

Honey (optional, for sweetness)

Instructions:

Combine all the ingredients in a blender.

Blend until smooth.

Add honey if desired for sweetness.

## Quinoa-Stuffed Bell Peppers:

Ingredients:

4 bell peppers (any color)

1 cup quinoa, rinsed

1 can black beans, drained and rinsed

1 can diced tomatoes (with juice)

1 cup of corn kernels (you can use fresh, frozen, or canned)

1 teaspoon chili powder

1/2 teaspoon cumin

Salt and pepper to taste

Grated cheese (optional, for topping)

**Instructions:**

Preheat your oven to 375°F (190°C).

Trim the tops of the bell peppers and scoop out the seeds and membranes.

In a large bowl, combine quinoa, black beans, diced tomatoes, corn, chili powder, cumin, salt, and pepper.

Place the bell pepper with the quinoa mixture.

Put the stuffed peppers in a baking dish and cover them with aluminum foil.

Then bake for 35-40 minutes or until the peppers are are boiled

If desired, sprinkle grated cheese on top and bake for an additional 5 minutes until melted.

Conclusion

A nutrient-rich meal plan tailored to the specific needs of individuals with bipolar disorder can help stabilize mood, improve overall well-being, and complement other treatment methods. Remember that dietary changes should be made in consultation with healthcare professionals to ensure they are safe and appropriate for your unique needs and circumstances. By prioritizing balanced nutrition, individuals with bipolar disorder can take important steps towards a more stable and fulfilling life.

## Schizophrenia

Schizophrenia is a complex and often misunderstood mental disorder characterized by symptoms such as hallucinations, delusions, disorganized thinking, and social withdrawal. While medication and therapy remain the primary treatments for schizophrenia, recent research has shed light on the potential role of nutrition in managing this condition. In this article, we will explore the relationship between nutrition and schizophrenia, examining how dietary choices and supplements can support individuals in their journey towards improved mental health and well-being.

The Schizophrenia-Nutrition Connection

1. **Omega-3 Fatty Acids:** Omega-3 fatty acids, commonly found in fatty fish like salmon, mackerel, and walnuts, have garnered attention for their potential role in managing schizophrenia. Studies suggest that omega-3 supplementation may reduce the severity of symptoms and improve cognitive function in individuals with schizophrenia. These essential fats have anti-inflammatory properties and may positively influence brain structure and function.

2. **Micronutrients:** Inadequacies in specific vitamins and minerals, including vitamin D, vitamin B12, folate,

and zinc, have been linked to an increased risk of schizophrenia and exacerbated symptoms. Ensuring an adequate intake of these nutrients through diet or supplements can be beneficial for managing this condition.

3. **Antioxidants:** Antioxidants, such as vitamin C, vitamin E, and selenium, can assist in shielding the brain from oxidative stress, a factor that has been implicated in schizophrenia. Including foods rich in antioxidants, like citrus fruits, nuts, and vegetables, may have a protective effect.

4. **Balanced Diet:** A well-balanced diet that provides essential nutrients, complex carbohydrates, and lean proteins is crucial for individuals with schizophrenia. Nutrient-rich foods support overall health and may contribute to symptom management.

5. **Gut Health:** The gut-brain connection is an emerging area of research, and imbalances in gut microbiota may play a role in schizophrenia. Consuming foods that support a healthy gut, such as fiber, fermented foods, and prebiotics, may have a positive impact on mental health.

6. **Caffeine and Alcohol:** Stimulants like caffeine and alcohol can exacerbate the symptoms of schizophrenia by disrupting sleep patterns and increasing agitation. Reducing or eliminating the consumption of these substances is recommended.

Challenges in Dietary Management of Schizophrenia

While nutrition can play a supportive role in managing schizophrenia, several challenges should be considered:

1. **Medication Interactions:** Many individuals with schizophrenia are prescribed antipsychotic medications that can affect appetite and metabolism. Some dietary choices and supplements may interact with these medications, emphasizing the need for healthcare provider guidance.

2. **Cognitive Impairments:** Cognitive deficits are common in schizophrenia, which can make it challenging for individuals to plan and maintain a nutritious diet. Support from family members, caregivers, or healthcare professionals may be necessary.

3. **Psychosocial Factors:** Individuals with schizophrenia may face social and economic challenges that impact their ability to access and afford nutritious foods. These barriers need to be addressed to ensure a well-rounded diet.

Sample Schizophrenia-Friendly Meal Plan

**Breakfast:**

- **Omega-3 Breakfast Bowl:** Top Greek yogurt with fresh berries, flaxseeds (for omega-3s), and a drizzle of honey for a nutritious and schizophrenia-friendly start to the day.

**Mid-Morning Snack:**

- **Mixed Nuts:** A small handful of mixed nuts provides healthy fats and protein, which can help maintain stable energy levels.

**Lunch:**

- **Salmon and Spinach Salad:** Grill or bake salmon and serve it over a bed of fresh spinach, cherry tomatoes, and a lemon vinaigrette for a nutrient-rich and schizophrenia-friendly lunch.

**Afternoon Snack:**

- **Sliced Bell Peppers with Hummus:** Bell peppers are rich in vitamin C, and hummus provides protein and healthy fats, making this a balanced and convenient snack.

**Dinner:**

- **Quinoa and Chickpea Stir-Fry:** Stir-fry quinoa with chickpeas, mixed vegetables, and a flavorful sauce for a wholesome and schizophrenia-friendly dinner.

**Dessert (if desired):**

- **Dark Chocolate**: A small piece of dark chocolate can satisfy sweet cravings without causing blood sugar spikes.

Conclusion

While nutrition is not a standalone treatment for schizophrenia, it can be a valuable complementary approach to help manage and alleviate the symptoms of this challenging mental disorder. A balanced diet rich in omega-3 fatty acids, micronutrients, antioxidants, and foods that support gut health, along with attention to blood sugar regulation and the avoidance of mood-altering substances, can contribute to improved mental health and overall well-being for individuals with schizophrenia. However, it is essential for individuals to work closely with their healthcare providers to tailor their dietary strategies to their unique needs and circumstances as part of a comprehensive treatment plan. By prioritizing balanced nutrition, individuals with schizophrenia can take important steps towards a more stable and fulfilling life.

## Stroke

Stroke is a life-altering medical event that occurs when there is a sudden disruption in blood flow to the brain, leading to the death of brain cells. The aftermath of a stroke can be physically and emotionally challenging, requiring a comprehensive approach to recovery. While medical intervention and rehabilitation are essential components of stroke management, emerging research suggests that nutrition plays a crucial role in aiding recovery and preventing future strokes. In this article, we will delve into the connection between nutrition and stroke, exploring how dietary choices can support individuals in their journey toward a healthier, post-stroke life.

The Stroke-Nutrition Connection

1. **Reducing Hypertension:** High blood pressure (hypertension) is a significant risk factor for stroke. A diet low in sodium (salt) and high in potassium, found in foods like bananas, leafy greens, and potatoes, can help regulate

blood pressure, reducing the risk of stroke.

2. **Anti-Inflammatory Foods:** Chronic inflammation can contribute to the development of atherosclerosis (hardening of the arteries), a leading cause of stroke. Foods rich in antioxidants, such as berries, nuts, and leafy greens, can help combat inflammation and protect blood vessels.

3. **Omega-3 Fatty Acids:** Omega-3 fatty acids, found in fatty fish like salmon and mackerel, have anti-inflammatory properties and can help reduce the risk of blood clots, which are often responsible for stroke.

4. **Fiber and Whole Grains:** Consuming a diet rich in fiber and whole grains can help control cholesterol levels and maintain a healthy weight, reducing the risk of atherosclerosis and stroke. Oats,

whole wheat, and brown rice are excellent choices.

5. **Maintaining a Healthy Weight:** A balanced diet combined with portion control and regular physical activity can help individuals achieve and maintain a healthy weight.

6. **Limiting Saturated and Trans Fats:** Foods high in saturated and trans fats, such as fried foods and baked goods, can contribute to the buildup of artery-clogging plaque. Reducing the consumption of these fats is essential for stroke prevention.

7. **Hydration:** Staying adequately hydrated is crucial for overall health and can help prevent blood clots. Drinking plenty of water and consuming hydrating foods like watermelon and cucumber can support stroke prevention.

8. **Alcohol Moderation:** Excessive alcohol consumption can increase blood pressure and contribute to stroke risk.

Challenges in Dietary Management Post-Stroke

While nutrition can significantly aid in stroke management, several challenges should be considered:

- Dysphagia: Many stroke survivors experience difficulty swallowing (dysphagia), which can affect their ability to eat certain foods. A speech therapist or dietitian can help design an appropriate diet plan that addresses these challenges.
- Medication Interactions: Some stroke survivors may be prescribed medications that interact with certain nutrients or dietary choices. Consulting with healthcare providers is crucial to ensure dietary adjustments do not interfere with medication dressing and

emotional aspects of nutrition is essential for long-term health.

Sample Post-Stroke Dietary Plan

A balanced post-stroke dietary plan should focus on nutrient-dense foods that support recovery and stroke prevention. Here is a sample meal plan:

## Breakfast:

Oatmeal topped with fresh berries and a sprinkle of flaxseeds for added fiber and omega-3 fatty acids.

A glass of potassium-rich banana and spinach smoothie.

Mid-Morning Snack:

Greek yogurt with honey and almonds for protein and antioxidants.

## Lunch:

Grilled salmon with a side of quinoa and steamed broccoli, providing omega-3s, protein, and fiber.

leafy green salad with a vinaigrette is nutritional

Afternoon Snack:

Sliced cucumber and carrot sticks with hummus for hydration and antioxidants.

## Dinner:

Baked chicken breast with a side of brown rice and sautéed spinach.

A fruit salad for dessert, such as watermelon and pineapple, to aid hydration.

Evening Snack (if needed):

A small handful of mixed nuts for healthy fats and protein.

While nutrition alone cannot prevent or cure stroke, it is an essential component of recovery and prevention. Adopting a diet that emphasizes whole, nutrient-dense foods, supports healthy weight management, and addresses risk factors like hypertension and inflammation can significantly aid in stroke management and reduce the risk of recurrent strokes. Stroke survivors should work closely with healthcare providers and dietitians to develop personalized dietary strategies that align with their specific needs and circumstances, ultimately contributing to a healthier and more fulfilling life post-stroke.

## Epilepsy

Epilepsy is a disease shown, medically affecting millions of people globally. While medications and other therapies remain the primary treatments for epilepsy, there is growing interest in how nutrition can complement these approaches and help individuals manage their condition more effectively. In this article, we will delve into the relationship between nutrition and epilepsy, exploring how dietary choices and strategies can play a significant role in seizure control and overall well-being.

## Understanding Epilepsy and Its Complexity

Epilepsy is a complex neurological condition where abnormal electrical activity in the brain leads to recurrent seizures. These seizures can vary widely in type and severity, making epilepsy a diverse disorder.

Managing epilepsy often involves identifying seizure triggers, medication management, and, increasingly, attention to dietary interventions.

## The Ketogenic Diet: A Powerful Tool for Seizure Control

One of the most well-known dietary approaches for managing epilepsy is the ketogenic diet. This high-fat, low-carbohydrate diet forces the body into a state of ketosis, where it primarily burns fat for energy.

The ketogenic diet has shown remarkable success in reducing seizure frequency, particularly in drug-resistant epilepsy cases. While the exact mechanisms are still under investigation, it is believed that ketones, produced during ketosis, have an anti-seizure effect on the brain.

Implementing the ketogenic diet involves strict adherence to macronutrient ratios.

With approximately 70-80% of calories coming from fat, 10-20% from protein, and 5-10% from carbohydrates. This approach requires careful planning and monitoring, often under the guidance of a healthcare professional or dietitian.

## Other Dietary Strategies for Epilepsy Management

- Modified Atkins Diet: Similar to the ketogenic diet but less restrictive in carbohydrate intake, the modified Atkins diet has been found to be effective in reducing seizure frequency. It is more manageable for many individuals because it allows for more carbohydrate consumption.
- Low Glycemic Index (GI) Diet: This diet focuses on consuming foods with a low glycemic index, which means they have a slower impact on blood sugar levels. Stable blood sugar can help reduce seizure frequency in some cases.
- Gluten-Free and Dairy-Free Diet: Some individuals with epilepsy may have sensitivities to gluten or dairy, which can trigger seizures in sensitive

individuals. Identifying and eliminating these trigger foods can help manage epilepsy.

- Fasting and Intermittent Fasting: Controlled fasting periods or intermittent fasting may mimic the effects of a ketogenic diet and promote ketosis. However, fasting should only be undertaken under the guidance of a healthcare professional.

- Supplements: Certain supplements, such as vitamin B6, magnesium, and omega-3 fatty acids, have shown potential in reducing seizure frequency. However, supplementation should be approached cautiously and under medical supervision.

**Challenges and Considerations**

While dietary interventions can be powerful tools in epilepsy management, they come with challenges:

Strict Adherence: Many dietary approaches for epilepsy require strict adherence to specific macronutrient ratios or the elimination of certain foods. This can be challenging and may require support from a dietitian or healthcare provider.

Nutrient Deficiencies: Some diets, like the ketogenic diet, may result in nutrient deficiencies over time. Proper supplementation and monitoring are crucial to prevent deficiencies.

Individual Variability: Epilepsy is highly individualized, and what is effective for one individual might not be suitable for someone else. Personalized dietary strategies are essential.

Medication Interactions: Dietary interventions may interact with epilepsy medications. It is essential to consult with a healthcare provider or dietitian to ensure compatibility.

Nutrition can be a valuable and complementary approach to managing epilepsy. While the ketogenic diet has gained significant attention for its potential in seizure control, other dietary strategies, such as low-GI diets, fasting, and eliminating trigger foods, should not be overlooked. Individuals with epilepsy should work closely with healthcare professionals and dietitians to develop personalized dietary plans that align with their specific needs and circumstances. With careful planning and monitoring, nutrition can play a vital role in helping individuals with epilepsy achieve better seizure control and overall well-being.

Meal plan and recipes for epilepsy

A ketogenic diet is often recommended as a therapeutic option for people with epilepsy, especially when other treatments have been ineffective. The ketogenic diet is a dietary approach characterized by its high-fat, low-carbohydrate, and moderate-protein composition, designed to can help control seizures in some individuals. However, it's essential to consult with a healthcare professional or a registered dietitian before embarking any diet for epilepsy, as they can provide personalized guidance and monitor your progress.

Here's a sample meal plan and some ketogenic recipes suitable for epilepsy management:

**Day 1:**

**Breakfast:**

- Eggs cooked in butter or coconut oil

- Avocado slices

- Spinach sautéed in olive oil

**Lunch:**

- Grilled chicken breast accompanied by a serving of steamed broccoli

- Caesar salad with high-fat dressing (made with olive oil and Parmesan)

**Snack:**

- Handful of macadamia nuts or almonds

**Dinner:**

- Salmon with a lemon and butter sauce

- Roasted asparagus with olive oil and Parmesan

- Mixed greens salad with an oil-based dressing

**Day 2:**

**Breakfast:**

- Keto-friendly smoothie with unsweetened almond milk, spinach, avocado, and a scoop of MCT oil or nut butter

**Lunch:**

- Ground beef or turkey lettuce wraps
  with guacamole and salsa

**Snack:**

- Celery sticks paired with either cream
  cheese or almond butter

**Dinner:**

- Pork chops with a creamy mushroom
  sauce (made with heavy cream)

- Steamed cauliflower mashed with
  butter and garlic

**Day 3:**

**Breakfast:**

- Full-fat Greek yogurt with a few berries
  and a drizzle of honey (if desired)

**Lunch:**

- Tuna salad prepared using canned tuna,
  mayonnaise, and diced celery, served in
  lettuce cups

**Snack:**

- Cheese slices or cheese sticks

**Dinner:**

- Beef or chicken stir-fry with low-carb vegetables (bell peppers, broccoli, and mushrooms) sautéed in coconut oil and soy sauce.

**Day 4:**

**Breakfast:**

- Omelet with cheese, diced bacon, and diced bell peppers

**Lunch:**

- Keto-friendly chicken or tuna salad with lots of mayo and greens

**Snack:**

- Hard-boiled eggs

**Dinner:**

Grilled shrimp served with a garlic and butter sauce

• Sautéed spinach prepared with olive oil and garlic

**Day 5:**

**Breakfast:**

- Keto pancakes made with almond flour and sugar-free syrup

**Lunch:**

- Roasted beef or turkey wrapped around cream cheese and pickles

**Snack:**

- Avocado with salt and pepper

**Dinner:**

- Baked cod featuring a pesto and Parmesan crust

- Roasted Brussels sprouts with bacon

Remember to drink plenty of water throughout the day, and it's advisable to consult with a healthcare professional or dietitian to ensure your specific dietary needs and macronutrient ratios align with your epilepsy management goals. Additionally, monitor your ketone levels to ensure you are in a state of ketosis, which is often the therapeutic goal of a ketogenic diet for epilepsy.

## Parkinson's Disease

Parkinson's Disease (PD) is a degenerative neurological condition that impacts millions of people worldwide. Characterized by symptoms such as tremors, bradykinesia(slowness of movement), muscle rigidity, and postural instability, PD significantly impacts a person's quality of life. While medications and therapies are primary treatments for PD, emerging research highlights the vital role of nutrition in managing symptoms and potentially slowing the progression of the disease. In this book, we will discuss the connection between nutrition and Parkinson's Disease, delving into how dietary choices and strategies can support individuals in their journey towards better health and well-being.

The Parkinson's-Nutrition Connection

1. **Antioxidants:** Oxidative stress and inflammation play a role in the progression of PD. Antioxidants, such as vitamins C and E, and polyphenols found in fruits, vegetables, and green tea, can help combat oxidative damage and reduce inflammation.

2. **Omega-3 Fatty Acids:** Omega-3 fatty acids, found in fatty fish, flaxseeds, and walnuts, possess anti-inflammatory properties that may be beneficial in reducing PD-related inflammation and improving brain health.

3. **Levodopa Absorption:** Levodopa, the primary medication used to manage PD symptoms, can have variable absorption rates when taken with food. Consuming a low-protein diet, especially in the morning when levodopa is typically taken, may help improve medication effectiveness.

4. **Balanced Diet:** A balanced diet rich in whole grains, lean proteins, fruits, and vegetables can help support overall health and manage PD symptoms.

5. **Hydration:** Dehydration can exacerbate muscle cramps and other PD symptoms. Staying well-hydrated is essential for managing PD.

6. **Probiotics and Gut Health:** There is emerging evidence linking gut health to PD. Consuming probiotics and foods rich in dietary fiber may support a healthy gut microbiome, potentially benefiting PD management.

7. **Vitamin D:** Vitamin D deficiency is common in PD and may contribute to muscle weakness and impaired balance. Ensuring an adequate intake of vitamin D through sunlight exposure and dietary sources can be beneficial.

Challenges in Dietary Management of Parkinson's Disease

While nutrition can be a valuable tool in managing PD, several challenges should be considered:

1. **Dysphagia:** Many individuals with PD experience difficulties with swallowing (dysphagia), which can affect their ability to eat certain foods. Speech therapists and dietitians can help design appropriate diet plans.

2. **Medication Timing:** PD medications must be taken at specific times and in coordination with meals. Managing

medication schedules alongside dietary plans can be complex.

3. **Individual Variability:** PD is highly individualized, and what works for one person may not work for another. Personalized dietary strategies are crucial.

4. **Interaction with Medications:** Some dietary choices or supplements may interact with PD medications. Consultation with healthcare providers is essential to ensure compatibility.

5. **Weight Management:** Weight loss or gain can be common in PD, impacting overall health. Sustaining an optimal weight via dietary choices and exercise is important.

Sample Parkinson's Disease Dietary Plan

A balanced dietary plan for someone with Parkinson's Disease should focus on nutrient-dense foods that support overall health and symptom management. Here is a sample meal plan:

**Breakfast:**

- Oatmeal topped with fresh berries and a sprinkle of chopped nuts (rich in antioxidants and fiber).

- A glass of orange juice (vitamin C source).

**Mid-Morning Snack:**

- Greek yogurt with honey and almonds (protein and antioxidants).

**Lunch:**

- Grilled chicken breast with a side of quinoa and steamed broccoli (lean protein, whole grains, and vegetables).

- A leafy green salad with a vinaigrette dressing (antioxidants).

**Afternoon Snack:**

- Sliced bell peppers and cucumber with hummus (hydration, fiber, and antioxidants).

**Dinner:**

- Baked salmon with brown rice and sautéed spinach (omega-3 fatty acids, whole grains, and leafy greens).

- Steamed asparagus (vitamins and fiber).

**Evening Snack (if needed):**

- A small handful of mixed nuts (healthy fats and protein).

Conclusion

While nutrition alone cannot cure Parkinson's Disease, it is an essential component of managing symptoms, improving overall health, and potentially slowing disease progression. A well-rounded nutritional plan abundant in antioxidants and omega-3, fatty acids, and nutrient-dense foods can support individuals in their journey toward better health and well-being. People with Parkinson's Disease should work closely with healthcare providers and dietitians to develop personalized dietary plans that align with their specific needs and circumstances. With careful planning and monitoring, nutrition can play a vital role in helping individuals with Parkinson's Disease achieve better symptom management and overall quality of life.

# Alzheimer's Disease

Alzheimer's Disease (AD) is a progressive neurodegenerative disorder Marked by a loss of memory, a decline in cognitive abilities, and alterations in behavior. Though Alzheimer's disease remains without a cure, recent studies indicate that nutrition plays a significant role in managing symptoms, slowing progression, and possibly diminishing the chances of encountering this debilitating ailment. Within this article, we will explore the link between dietary choices and Alzheimer's Disease, exploring how dietary choices and strategies can support individuals in their journey towards better cognitive health and well-being.

**The Alzheimer's-Nutrition Connection**

1. **Antioxidants: Oxidative stress and inflammation are implicated in the development and progression of Alzheimer's Disease. Antioxidants, such as vitamins C and E, and polyphenols found in fruits, vegetables, and green tea, can help combat oxidative damage and reduce inflammation.**

2. **Omega-3 Fatty Acids:** Omega-3 fatty acids, primarily found in fatty fish like salmon, mackerel, and flaxseeds, have anti-inflammatory properties and are

associated with improved cognitive function. Consuming these fats may help protect brain cells and reduce the risk of cognitive decline.

3. **Healthy Fats:** A diet rich in healthy fats, including monounsaturated fats (found in olive oil and avocados) and polyunsaturated fats (found in nuts and seeds), can support brain health and reduce the risk of cognitive impairment.

4. **Balanced Diet:** A diet that includes a variety of nutrient-dense foods, including items like fruits, vegetables, whole grains, lean sources of protein, and beneficial fats, provides essential vitamins and minerals that support overall cognitive function.

5. **Low Glycemic Index (GI) Foods:** Consuming low-GI foods, which have a slower impact on blood sugar levels, can help maintain stable energy levels

and may reduce the risk of cognitive decline.

6. **Vitamin D:** Adequate vitamin D intake is associated with improved cognitive function. Being in the sun and intake of vitamin D- rich foods like fatty fish and fortified dairy products can help support cognitive health.

7. **B Vitamins:** B vitamins, including B6, B12, and folate, are essential for brain health and may help reduce homocysteine levels in the blood, which is linked to cognitive decline.

## Challenges in Dietary Management of Alzheimer's Disease

While nutrition can play a significant role in Alzheimer's management, several challenges should be considered:

1. **Dysphagia:** Many individuals with Alzheimer's experience difficulties with swallowing (dysphagia), which can

affect their ability to eat certain foods. Speech therapists and dietitians can help design appropriate diet plans.

2. **Medication Interactions:** Some dietary choices or supplements may interact with medications used to manage Alzheimer's symptoms. Consultation with healthcare providers is essential to ensure compatibility.

3. **Individual Variability:** Alzheimer's Disease is highly individualized, and what's effective for one individual might not be suitable for someone else. Tailored or individualized dietary strategies are crucial.

4. **Weight Management:** Weight loss is common in Alzheimer's, impacting overall health. Sustaining an optimal body weight through dietary choices and physical activity is important.

# Sample Alzheimer's Disease Dietary Plan

A balanced dietary plan for someone with Alzheimer's Disease should focus on nutrient-dense foods that support overall cognitive health. Here is a sample meal plan:

**Breakfast:**

- Greek yogurt with fresh berries and a drizzle of honey (antioxidants and probiotics).

- Whole-grain toast with avocado (healthy fats and fiber).

**Mid-Morning Snack:**

- A small handful of walnuts (omega-3 fatty acids and antioxidants).

**Lunch:**

- Grilled chicken salad with mixed greens, cherry tomatoes, and a vinaigrette dressing (vitamins, minerals, and antioxidants).

- A side of quinoa (whole grains and protein).

**Afternoon Snack:**

- Sliced cucumber and carrot sticks with hummus (hydration, fiber, and antioxidants).

**Dinner:**

- Baked salmon with brown rice and steamed broccoli (omega-3 fatty acids, whole grains, and vegetables).

- Steamed asparagus (vitamins and fiber).

**Evening Snack (if needed):**

- A small piece of dark chocolate (antioxidants).

While nutrition alone cannot cure Alzheimer's Disease, it is an essential component of managing symptoms, slowing progression, and potentially reducing the risk of cognitive decline. A balanced diet rich in antioxidants, omega-3 fatty acids, healthy fats, and nutrient-dense foods can support individuals in their journey toward better cognitive health and well-being. People with Alzheimer's Disease should work closely with healthcare providers and dietitians to develop personalized dietary plans that align with their specific needs and circumstances. With careful planning and monitoring, nutrition can play a vital role in helping individuals with Alzheimer's Disease achieve better cognitive function and overall quality of life.

# Chapter 9

# Mindful Eating for
# Mental Wellness

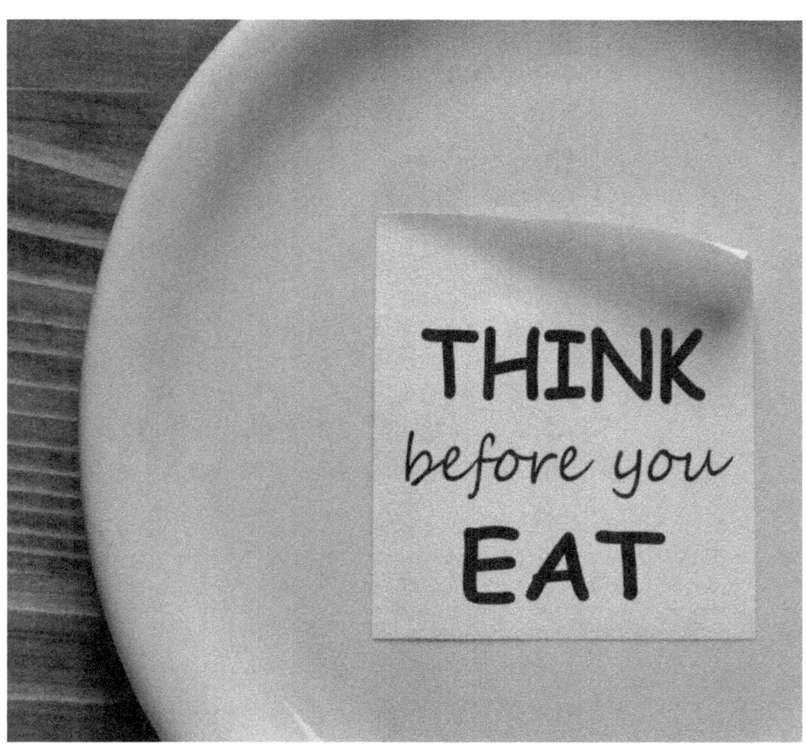

# The practice of mindful eating

In our fast-paced, modern world, it's easy to rush through meals, barely pausing to taste or appreciate the food we consume. Mindful eating, however, involves a habit that promotes mindfulness, urging us to take our time, stay in the moment, and relish each bite. Beyond just satisfying our hunger, mindful eating promotes a deeper connection with food, enhances our well-being, and fosters a healthier relationship with eating. Within this article, we will delve into the idea of practicing mindfulness in eating, its benefits, and how to incorporate this practice into your daily life.

What Is Mindful Eating?

Mindful eating is an ancient practice rooted in Buddhist teachings, which has gained popularity in recent years as a holistic approach to healthier eating habits. At its core, mindful eating is about paying full attention to the sensory experience of eating, including the taste, texture, aroma, and even the sound of food. It involves being present in the moment and making conscious choices about what, when, and how we eat.

The Principles of Mindful Eating

1. **Eat with Awareness:** Mindful eating begins with being aware of your food choices. This means acknowledging what you are about to eat and understanding its nutritional value and impact on your body.

2. **Engage All Senses:** As you eat, engage all your senses. Notice the colors, textures, and smells of your food. Pay attention to how it feels in your mouth and the flavors that unfold with each bite.

3. **Eat Slowly:** Avoid rushing through meals. Chew your food thoroughly.

Eating slowly allows your body to signal fullness more accurately, helping prevent overeating.

4. **Eliminate Distractions:** Minimize distractions during meals. Turn off the TV, put away your smartphone, and create a peaceful environment that allows you to focus on your food.

5. Pay attention to your body. Consume food when your body signals hunger and cease when you feel content, not when your plate is empty.

6. **Practice Gratitude:** Cultivate gratitude for the food you're consuming. Understand the effort and resources that went into producing your meal.

The Benefits of Mindful Eating

1. **Weight Management:** Mindful eating can help regulate portion sizes and prevent overeating, making it a valuable tool for weight management.

2. **Improved Digestion:** Chewing food slowly and thoroughly aids in digestion and reduces digestive discomfort.

3. **Enhanced Satisfaction:** By savoring each bite, you may find that smaller portions of well-enjoyed food satisfy you more than larger portions of hurriedly consumed meals.

4. **Stress Reduction:** Mindful eating can reduce stress and emotional eating by promoting relaxation and a sense of mindfulness.

5. **Better Food Choices:** Being more aware of your food choices can lead to healthier eating habits as you become attuned to your body's needs.

6. **Enhanced Enjoyment:** Mindful eating enhances the pleasure of eating, allowing you to savor the flavors and textures of food fully.

How to Incorporate Mindful Eating into Your
Life

1. **Start with Small Steps:** Begin by
   designating one meal or snack per day
   as your "mindful eating practice."
   Gradually, you can expand this to other
   meals.

2. **Create a Peaceful Environment:** Find
   a quiet and comfortable place to eat
   without distractions. Set a pleasing
   atmosphere with minimal clutter.

3. **Use All Your Senses:** Before taking a
   bite, take a moment to visually
   appreciate your food. Smell it, touch it,
   and observe its textures.

4. **Chew Slowly:** Make an effort to chew
   each bite thoroughly, savoring the
   flavors. Put your utensils down between
   bites.

5. **Practice Mindful Breathing:** Take
   deep breaths before, during, and after

your meal. This helps you stay present and connected to your eating experience.

6. **Listen to Your Body:** Eat in response to your hunger cues and halt your consumption when you feel satisfied.

7. **Reflect on Your Meal:** After finishing your meal, take a moment to reflect on your experience. What did you enjoy most about it? How did you feel physically and emotionally?

Conclusion

Mindful eating is not a diet; it's a way of cultivating a healthier, more satisfying relationship with food. By practicing mindfulness at mealtime, you can transform the act of eating into a mindful, pleasurable, and nourishing experience. Over time, this practice can lead to a deeper connection with your body's hunger and fullness signals, better food choices, and an overall sense of well-being. So, slow down, savor each bite, and relish the simple joy of nourishing your body and soul through mindful eating.

## Combining nutrition and mindfulness for better mental health

Mental health is a cornerstone of overall well-being, and its connection to nutrition and mindfulness has gained significant attention in recent years. As our understanding of holistic health grows, we increasingly recognize the profound impact that the food we consume and our mental state can have on each other. In this article, we will explore the powerful synergy of nutrition and mindfulness, and how their combination can contribute to better mental health.

The Mind-Nutrition Nexus

1. **The Gut-Brain Connection:** Emerging research has unveiled a strong

connection between the gut and the brain, known as the gut-brain axis. The composition of the gut microbiome, influenced by diet, can affect mental health. A balanced diet supports a healthy gut microbiome, potentially alleviating symptoms of anxiety and depression.

2. **Nutrient Deficiencies:** Inadequate intake of essential nutrients like omega-3 fatty acids, B vitamins, and antioxidants can negatively impact brain function. Nutrient-rich diets can help maintain cognitive health and reduce the risk of mental health disorders.

3. **Blood Sugar Regulation:** Fluctuations in blood sugar levels can influence mood swings and irritability. Consuming foods with a low glycemic index helps stabilize blood sugar, promoting emotional stability.

4. **Inflammation and Mood:** Chronic inflammation is associated with depression and other mental health issues. A diet rich in anti-inflammatory foods, such as fruits, vegetables, and fatty fish, can help mitigate inflammation.

Mindfulness for Mental Health

1. **Stress Alleviation:** Engaging in mindfulness techniques such as meditation and deep breathing exercises, can reduce stress levels. Chronic stress is a significant contributor to mental health problems.

2. **Emotion Regulation:** Mindfulness helps individuals observe their thoughts and emotions without judgment. This self-awareness can lead to improved emotional regulation and a reduction in symptoms of anxiety and depression.

3. **Enhanced Resilience:** Mindfulness can enhance psychological resilience, enabling individuals to more effectively manage life's difficulties and setbacks.

4. **Improved Sleep:** Mindfulness techniques promote better sleep, a crucial component of mental health. Inadequate sleep quality is associated with fluctuations in mood disorders and cognitive impairments.

5. **Greater Self-Acceptance:** Mindfulness fosters self-acceptance and self-compassion, reducing self-criticism and the risk of developing or aggravating mental health disorders such as eating disorders and body image issues.

Bringing Nutrition and Mindfulness Together

1. **Mindful Eating:** Combine the principles of mindfulness with your eating habits. Completely focus on the sensory

aspects of your meal while eating eating each bite, and appreciating the nourishment it provides. Don't watch TV or working on your computer while eat.

2. **Emotionally:**Mindfulness can help you pause and make more conscious decisions about what you eat, especially during moments of stress or emotional turmoil.

3. **Mindful Meal Planning:** When planning your meals, consider the nutritional content of your food and how it can support your mental health. Prioritize nutrient-dense foods and incorporate mood-boosting ingredients.

4. **Mindful Snacking:** Instead of mindlessly reaching for snacks, take a moment to assess your hunger and emotions. Choose snacks that satisfy your cravings and provide sustained energy, such as nuts or yogurt.

5. **Mindful Cooking:** Engage in the process of cooking with mindfulness, paying attention to the colors, textures, and aromas of the ingredients. Preparing meals can be a meditative experience that fosters a sense of calm.

Conclusion

The intertwining of nutrition and mindfulness holds the key to better mental health. By nourishing our bodies with balanced diets rich in essential nutrients, we support brain function and reduce the risk of mental health disorders. Simultaneously, practicing mindfulness can help us manage stress, regulate our emotions, and develop greater self-compassion. Combining these two powerful approaches allows us to cultivate a profound connection between our physical and mental well-being. Embrace the harmony of nourishment and awareness, and embark on a journey towards improved mental health and overall vitality.

# Chapter 10

## Balanced diet: A key to healthy living

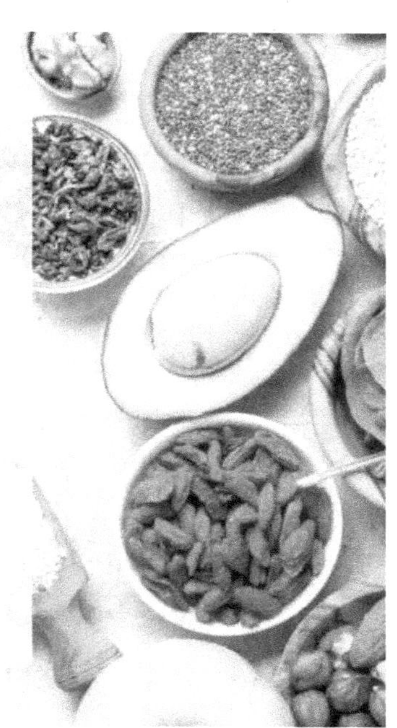

## A Balanced Diet for Life

# General dietary recommendations for mental well-being

In our pursuit of well-being, it's essential to recognize the profound impact of nutrition on our mental health. A balanced diet not only supports our physical health but also plays a pivotal role in nurturing a resilient and vibrant mind. The connection between nutrition and mental well-being is a subject of increasing research and understanding. In this comprehensive article, we will delve deeply into general dietary recommendations for mental well-being, exploring the science behind these guidelines and their practical application in our daily lives.

The Gut-Brain Connection

Before we embark on our exploration of dietary recommendations for mental well-being, it's crucial to understand the fascinating connection between our gut and brain. The gut-brain axis serves as a two-way communication network between the gut microbiota and the central nervous system. Emerging research suggests that the composition of our gut microbiome, influenced significantly by our diet, can have profound effects on mood, emotions, and mental health.

## 1. Balanced Macronutrients: The Foundation of Mental Wellness

A balanced diet is like a symphony of macronutrients (carbohydrates, proteins, and fats), each playing a unique role in supporting our mental well-being.

- **Carbohydrates:** Choose complex carbohydrates present in whole grains, fruits, and vegetables. These foods provide a steady source of glucose, the brain's primary fuel, which helps stabilize mood and energy levels.

- **Proteins:** Protein-rich foods like lean meats, fish, eggs, and legumes contain amino acids that serve as building blocks for neurotransmitters. These neurotransmitters, such as serotonin and dopamine, profoundly influence our mood and feelings of well-being.

- **Fats:** Incorporate healthy fats, particularly those rich in omega-3 fatty acids, found in fatty fish like salmon, nuts, seeds, and avocados. Omega-3s have been linked to reduced symptoms of depression and anxiety, enhancing overall mental wellness.

2. **Antioxidant-Rich Foods: Guardians of Mental Clarity**

Antioxidants are like the guardians of our brain cells, protecting them from oxidative stress, which can contribute to mood disorders and cognitive decline. A diet rich in antioxidants from colorful fruits and vegetables, nuts, and seeds helps keep our mental faculties sharp.

3. **Vitamins and Minerals: The Mental Health Superheroes**

Certain vitamins and minerals are mental health superheroes, ensuring our cognitive functions remain in top shape.

- **B Vitamins:** The B-vitamin family, including B6, B9 (folate), and B12, are pivotal for brain health. They participate in neurotransmitter production and can be found in foods like leafy greens, lean meats, and legumes.

- **Magnesium:** This mineral is essential for regulating mood and reducing symptoms of depression. There are various types of seeds Nuts-seeds, whole grains, and leafy greens

- **Zinc:** Inadequate zinc levels have been associated with mood disorders Sources include oysters, red meat, poultry, and beans.

4. **Hydration: The Fountain of Mental Clarity**

Dehydration can lead to cognitive impairment, mood disturbances, and increased stress. Staying adequately hydrated by drinking water throughout the day and consuming hydrating foods like fruits and vegetables is vital for mental well-being.

5. **Limit Processed and Sugary Foods: Mood's Silent Agitators**

Highly processed foods and excessive sugar consumption have been associated with an increased risk of mood disorders and cognitive decline. Limiting your intake of sugary snacks, sugary beverages, and processed foods can significantly enhance mental wellness.

6. **Moderate Caffeine and Alcohol: Juggling Act for Mental Health**

Caffeine and alcohol can affect sleep patterns and mood. While moderate consumption may be acceptable for some, excessive intake can disrupt mental well-being. Mindful monitoring of your caffeine and alcohol intake can help maintain mental equilibrium.

### 7. **Omega-3 Fatty Acids: Brain's Nutrient-Rich Fuel**

Fatty fish like salmon, mackerel, and sardines are rich sources of omega-3 fatty acids, known as the brain's nutrient-rich fuel. These essential fats are linked to improved mood and reduced symptoms of depression and anxiety. If fish consumption isn't regular, considering omega-3 supplements can be beneficial.

### 8. **Probiotics and Gut Health: The Mood's Microbiome Managers**

Cutting-edge research highlights the intimate connection between gut health and mental well-being. Incorporating probiotic-rich foods like yogurt, kefir, and sauerkraut supports a healthy gut microbiome, potentially benefiting mood and mental resilience.

## 9. Mindful Eating: The Gateway to Mental Nourishment

Beyond the specifics of what we eat, how we eat holds profound importance. The practice of mindful eating encourages us to be fully present during meals, fostering a deeper connection between our mind and nourishment.

**Mindful Eating Principles:**

**Present Awareness: Be fully present during meals, acknowledging the act of eating and savoring each bite.**

**Engage All Senses: Utilize your senses to appreciate the experience fully. Listen to the sounds of your meal, and savor the evolving flavors with each bite.**

Chew Slowly: Avoid rushing through meals. Take the time to chew your food thoroughly, allowing your body to signal fullness more accurately and preventing overeating.

Minimize Distractions: Establish a serene dining setting by reducing distractions. Switch off the television, and stow away your smartphone, and focus solely on your meal.

Tune into Your Body: Be mindful of signals for hunger and satiety. Consume food when you feel hungry and discontinue when you sense satisfaction, rather than when your plate is empty.

Practice Gratitude: Develop a sense of gratitude for the food you consume. Understand the effort and resources that went into producing your meal, fostering appreciation for the nourishment it provides.

## Conclusion

Nutrition is a cornerstone of mental well-being, and understanding the symbiotic relationship between what we eat and how we feel is paramount. These general dietary recommendations, informed by scientific research and the principles of mindful eating, provide a holistic approach to nurturing your mental wellness. By embracing these guidelines and applying them in your daily life, you embark on a journey toward a happier, more emotionally resilient, and mentally vibrant existence. Remember that while nutrition is a powerful ally in your pursuit of mental well-being, it should complement other self-care practices, such as regular exercise, adequate sleep, and seeking professional help when needed. Nourish both your body and mind, and watch as your mental well-being blossoms into a state of vitality and equilibrium.

# CONCLUSION

# The role of food in mental health

The significance of nutrition in mental health is a subject of growing interest and research. Beyond satisfying hunger, the food we consume has a profound impact on our cognitive function, mood regulation, and overall mental well-being. The relationship between diet and mental health is intricate and multifaceted, with a burgeoning body of evidence highlighting the vital role food plays in nurturing a sound mind. In this comprehensive article, we will delve deeply into the intricate interplay between nutrition and mental health, exploring the science behind this connection and providing practical insights into how you can harness the power of food to support and optimize your mental well-being.

The Brain's Nutritional Demands

The human brain, a remarkably complex organ, is the epicenter of our thoughts, emotions, and behaviors. To function optimally, it requires a consistent supply of energy and essential nutrients. These nutrients serve as building blocks for neurotransmitters, the chemical messengers that facilitate communication between brain cells, influencing our mood, cognitive abilities, and overall mental health.

## 1. **Glucose: Fuel for the Brain**

Glucose, derived from carbohydrates, is the brain's primary source of energy. It fuels cognitive functions, such as decision-making, memory, and problem-solving. A diet rich in complex carbohydrates, like whole grains, fruits, and vegetables, provides a steady supply of glucose, ensuring the brain's energy demands are met without the rollercoaster of blood sugar spikes and crashes.

## 2. **Proteins: Amino Acids for Neurotransmitters**

Proteins, composed of amino acids, are essential for neurotransmitter production. Neurotransmitters like serotonin, dopamine, and norepinephrine profoundly influence mood and emotional well-being. Consuming adequate protein sources, including lean meats, fish, eggs, and legumes, supports the synthesis of these vital neurotransmitters.

## 3. **Fats:Omega-3s and Cognitive Health**

Healthy fats, particularly omega-3 fatty acids found in fatty fish (e.g., salmon, mackerel), walnuts, flaxseeds, and chia seeds, are crucial for maintaining cognitive function and reducing the risk of mental health disorders.

Omega-3s contribute to the structure of brain cell membranes and promote neuroplasticity, the brain's ability to adapt and reorganize.

## 4. Micronutrients: Vitamins and Minerals for Brain Health

Micronutrients like vitamins and minerals play a pivotal role in maintaining brain health and mental well-being:

- **B Vitamins:** Essential B vitamins such as B6, B9 (folate), and B12 for neurotransmitter production and overall cognitive function. Deficiencies in these vitamins have been linked to mood disorders and cognitive decline.

- **Vitamin D:** Adequate vitamin D levels are associated with improved mood and reduced risk of depression. Exposure to sunlight and consumption of vitamin D-rich foods, like fatty fish and fortified dairy products, support mental well-being.

- **Magnesium:** This mineral is crucial for regulating mood and reducing symptoms of depression. Foods rich in magnesium include nuts, seeds, whole grains, and leafy greens.

- **Zinc:** Zinc plays a role in neurotransmitter function and mood regulation. Oysters, red meat, poultry, and beans are excellent sources.

- **Antioxidants:** Antioxidants, such as vitamins C and E, protect brain cells from oxidative stress, which can contribute to mood disorders and cognitive decline. Fruits, vegetables, nuts, and seeds are rich sources of antioxidants.

## Nutrition and Mental Health: A Bidirectional Relationship

While the right nutrients nourish the brain and support mental health, mental health itself can significantly impact dietary choices.

Stress, anxiety, and depression can lead to changes in appetite, food preferences, and eating habits.

## The Gut-Brain Connection

Beyond the nutritional aspects, the gut-brain connection is an emerging field of research shedding light on how the gut microbiome influences mental health.

The gut microbiome, a diverse community of microorganisms residing in the digestive tract, communicates with the brain through the gut-brain axis.

Mood and Microbes: Research suggests that an imbalance in the gut microbiome, known as dysbiosis, may contribute to mood disorders like depression and anxiety. A diet rich in fiber and prebiotic foods, such as fruits, vegetables, and fermented foods like yogurt and kimchi, supports a diverse and healthy gut microbiome, potentially benefiting mental well-being.

Inflammation and Mental Health: Chronic inflammation has been linked to depression and other mental health issues. Consuming anti-inflammatory foods, including fruits, vegetables, fatty fish, and spices like turmeric, can help mitigate inflammation and support mental wellness.

The Mediterranean Diet: A Blueprint for Mental Health

The Mediterranean diet, renowned for its positive impact on cardiovascular health, is emerging as a dietary pattern that also supports mental well-being. This diet emphasizes nutrient-rich foods, such as:

Fruits and Vegetables: Abundant in antioxidants, vitamins, and minerals that protect the brain from oxidative stress and support cognitive function.

Fatty Fish: A regular intake of fish like salmon, mackerel, and sardines provides omega-3 fatty acids, which have been associated with reduced symptoms of depression and anxiety.

OliveOil:

Abundant in monounsaturated fats and antioxidants, olive oil promotes brain health and diminishes the likelihood of cognitive decline.

Nuts and Seeds: Walnuts, almonds, flaxseeds, and chia seeds provide healthy fats, fiber, and essential nutrients that promote cognitive function and mental well-being.

Legumes: Beans, lentils, and chickpeas serve as superb protein sources fiber, and B vitamins, contributing to neurotransmitter production and mood regulation.

Whole Grains: Whole grains like quinoa, brown rice, and whole wheat pasta offer complex carbohydrates that provide sustained energy and stabilize mood.

**Herbs and Spices:** Herbs like rosemary and basil, as well as spices like turmeric, offer anti-inflammatory and antioxidant properties that support brain health.

Red Wine (in moderation): Some studies suggest that moderate red wine consumption may be linked to a reduced risk of depression and cognitive decline due to its antioxidant content.

## Empowerment Through Dietary Choices

Empowerment in the realm of diet and mental wellness involves making informed choices, cultivating a positive relationship with food, and recognizing the agency we possess to shape our well-being.

1. Educate Yourself: Knowledge is Empowerment

The journey begins with knowledge. Educate yourself about the profound impact of diet on mental health. Understand the role of macronutrients, micronutrients, and dietary patterns in fostering emotional resilience and cognitive clarity.

**Seek Professional Guidance: A Path to Informed Choices**

Empowerment embraces the wisdom of seeking professional guidance when needed. If you have specific dietary concerns or mental health issues, consider consulting with a registered dietitian or mental health professional who specializes in nutrition.

Taking charge of your diet and mental wellness is not a journey for the faint-hearted; it is a journey for those who recognize the incredible power they hold to shape their well-being. The interplay between diet and mental wellness is a profound testament to our capacity for transformation.

It is an affirmation that with knowledge, mindfulness, and balanced choices, we can empower ourselves to nurture emotional resilience, enhance cognitive function, and cultivate a profound sense of well-being.

As you embark on this transformative journey, remember that empowerment thrives on education, mindfulness, and balance. Cultivate a positive relationship with food, embrace the agency you possess to shape your well-being, and recognize the profound impact your choices have on your mental health. In the end, it is not just about nourishing your body; it is about nourishing your mind, heart, and soul, forging a path toward a life marked by vitality, equilibrium, and unwavering mental wellness.